THE
HEART HEALTHY
COOKBOOK FOR BEGINNERS

1800 Days of Easy & Flavorful Low-Sodium, Low-Fat Recipes to Maintain Blood Pressure and Enjoy Healthy Living. Includes 60-Day Meal Plan & 2 Bonuses

Susan Elliott

ISBN: 9798392831128

TABLE OF CONTENTS

INTRODUCTION 6

FOOD TO AVOID 7

FOOD TO EAT 9

BENEFITS OF HEART HEALTHY DIETS
.... 10

BEANS, GRAINS AND PASTA 12

Small Pasta and Beans Pot 12

Wild Rice, Celery, and Cauliflower Pilaf 12

Minestrone Chickpeas and Macaroni Casserole
.... 13

Slow Cooked Turkey and Brown Rice 13

Papaya, Jicama, and Peas Rice Bowl 14

Italian Baked Beans 14

Cannellini Bean Lettuce Wraps 14

Israeli Eggplant, Chickpea, and Mint Sauté 15

Lentils and Rice 16

Brown Rice Pilaf with Pistachios and Raisins 16

Cherry, Apricot, and Pecan Brown Rice Bowl
.... 17

Curry Apple Couscous with Leeks and Pecans
.... 17

Lebanese Flavor Broken Thin Noodles 17

Lemony Farro and Avocado Bowl 18

Rice and Blueberry Stuffed Sweet Potatoes ... 18

Farrotto Mix 19

Feta-Grape-Bulgur Salad with Grapes and Feta
.... 19

Greek Style Meaty Bulgur 20

Hearty Barley Mix.................................. 20

Hearty Barley Risotto 21

Hearty Freekeh Pilaf 22

Herby-Lemony Farro 22

Mushroom-Bulgur Pilaf 23

Baked Brown Rice 23

Barley Pilaf 24

Basmati Rice Pilaf Mix 24

Brown Rice Salad with Asparagus, Goat Cheese,
and Lemon 25

Carrot-Almond-Bulgur Salad 25

Chickpea-Spinach-Bulgur 26

Greek Farro Salad................................. 26

POULTRY AND MEAT RECIPES 27

Lemon-Garlic Chicken and Green Beans with
Caramelized Onions............................ 27

Tarragon Chicken with Roasted Balsamic
Turnips 27

Turmeric Chicken Wings with Ginger Sauce . 28

Curry Chicken Lettuce Wraps 28

Nacho Chicken Casserole 28

Pesto & Mozzarella Chicken Casserole.......... 29

Chicken Quiche 29

Chicken Parmigiana............................... 30

Baked Chicken Meatballs - Habanero & Green
Chili 30

Winter Chicken with Vegetables 31

Paprika Chicken & Pancetta in a Skillet.......... 31

Chili & Lemon Marinated Chicken Wings 31

Cipollini & Bell Pepper Chicken Souvlaki...... 32

Pulled Buffalo Chicken Salad with Blue Cheese
.... 32

Red Pepper and Mozzarella-Stuffed Chicken
Caprese 33

Turnip Greens & Artichoke Chicken.............. 33

VEGETABLES AND VEGAN RECIPES... 34

Lentils with Tomatoes and Turmeric............. 34

Whole-Wheat Pasta with Tomato-Basil Sauce
.... 34

Nutty and Fruity Garden Salad 35

Roasted Root Vegetables...................................35

Braised Kale..35

Braised Leeks, Cauliflower and Artichoke Hearts 36

Celery Root Hash Browns 36

Braised Carrots 'n Kale 36

Cauliflower Fritters..37

Sweet Potato Puree 37

Vegetable Potpie..38

Fruit Bowl with Yogurt Topping...................38

Collard Green Wrap..39

Wild Rice with Spicy Chickpeas 39

Mashed Cauliflower...40

Cashew Pesto & Parsley with veggies 40

Spicy Chickpeas with Roasted Vegetables......41

Special Vegetable Kitchree...............................41

Mashed Sweet Potato Burritos 41

Toasted Cumin Crunch 42

Light Mushroom Risotto.................................42

Vegetable Pie...43

Turmeric Nachos...43

Rucola Salad 44

Tasty Spring Salad 44

Pure Delish Spinach Salad...............................44

FISH AND SEAFOOD RECIPES.............45

Lemon-Caper Trout with Caramelized Shallots 45

Manhattan-Style Salmon Chowder 45

Roasted Salmon and Asparagus 46

Citrus Salmon on a Bed of Greens.................46

Orange and Maple-Glazed Salmon.................47

Salmon Ceviche 47

Cod with Ginger and Black Beans..................48

Rosemary-Lemon Cod.....................................48

Halibut Curry 48

Baked Tomato Hake..49

Salmon and Roasted Peppers 49

Shrimp and Beets...50

Shrimp and Corn 50

Poached Halibut and Mushrooms 50

Halibut Stir Fry 51

Steamed Garlic-Dill Halibut 51

Italian Halibut Chowder..................................52

Dill Haddock...52

Honey Crusted Salmon with Pecans 52

Salmon and Cauliflower...................................53

Ginger Salmon and Black Beans.....................53

Cod Curry 54

Healthy Fish Nacho Bowl...............................54

Fish & Chickpea Stew......................................54

Easy Crunchy Fish Tray Bake 55

Ginger & Chili Sea Bass Fillets.......................55

Nut-Crust Tilapia with Kale 56

Wasabi Salmon Burgers...................................56

Citrus & Herb Sardines 57

Spicy Kingfish 57

Gingered Tilapia 58

Haddock with Swiss chard...............................58

Coconut Rice with shrimps in Coconut curry 58

Herbed Rockfish..59

Stuffed Trout...59

Thai Chowder..60

Seared Ahi Tuna 60

Quick Shrimp Moqueca...................................61

Souvlaki Spiced Salmon Bowls........................61

Prosciutto-Wrapped Haddock.........................62

Grilled Salmon with Caponata 62

Herbed Coconut Milk Steamed Mussels.........63

Basil Halibut Red Pepper Packets 64

Oven-Baked Sole Fillets 64

Keto Oodles with White Clam Sauce 64

Fried Codfish with Almonds 65

Salmon Balls 65

Codfish Sticks 66

Lemony Trout 66

Quick Fish Bowl 66

Tender Creamy Scallops 67

Salmon Cakes 67

Salmon with Mustard Cream 68

Tuna Steaks with Shirataki Noodles 68

Tilapia with Parmesan Bark 69

Blackened Fish Tacos with Slaw 69

AIR FRYER (BONUS) 70

Air Fryer Chicken Tacos 70

Air Fryer Tofu Stir Fry 71

Air Fryer Breakfast Burritos 72

Air Fryer Mushroom Risotto 72

Air Fryer Meatball Subs 73

Air Fryer Fried Rice 74

Air Fryer Coconut Chicken 75

Air Fryer Falafel Pitas 75

Air Fryer Chicken Nuggets 76

Air Fryer Salmon with Roasted Vegetables 77

Air Fryer Zucchini Fritters 77

Air Fryer Lemon Garlic Shrimp 78

FRUIT AND DESERT RECIPES 80

Chia and Berries Smoothie Bowl 80

Almond Butter Smoothies 80

Blended Coconut Milk and Banana Breakfast Smoothie 80

Kale Smoothie 80

Raspberry Smoothie 81

Pineapple Smoothie 81

Beet Smoothie 81

Blueberry Smoothie 81

Strawberry Oatmeal Smoothie 82

Almond Blueberry Smoothie 82

Raspberry Banana Smoothie 82

Avocado Chia Parfait 83

Pure Avocado Pudding 83

Sweet Almond and Coconut Fat Bombs 83

60 DAYS MEAL PLAN 85

GET YOUR BONUSES NOW 88

CONCLUSION 89

MEASUREMENT CONVERSION CHART 91

INTRODUCTION

Welcome to the Heart-Healthy Cookbook!

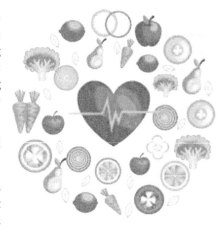

The health and happiness you experience in life are directly tied to the condition of your heart, one of the most critical organs in your body. It continuously beats throughout the day, pumping oxygen-rich blood to your brain and other body components. The health of your heart is closely tied to your overall well-being, and making the right choices about what you eat is one of the most critical steps to keep it in tip-top shape.

Heart-healthy foods are low in unhealthy fats, salt, and added sugars and high in nutrients like fibre, vitamins, and minerals.

It's vital to be aware that several recipes in this cookbook contain items such as high-fat meat, cheese, and oil, which may be detrimental to heart health if taken in excess. So, it's always good to be mindful of portion sizes and choose ingredients lower in unhealthy fats and added sugars.

These meals have been shown to aid in weight maintenance, decrease blood pressure as well as cholesterol, and lessen the danger of cardiovascular disease and stroke. There are a few examples of healthy foods for the heart that include:

Vegetables and Fruits:

These are packed with minerals, fibre, and vitamins and can help you stay full without consuming too many calories.

Fiber:

Fiber from whole grains is a fantastic source for lowering cholesterol and heart disease risk.

Lean proteins include foods like poultry, fish, and legumes and can help you build and repair muscle and provide essential nutrients like iron and B vitamins.

On the other hand, a heart-healthy diet also requires that you be aware of the items you ought to reduce or avoid. Among these are:

Saturated and Trans fats: High cholesterol and a higher chance of cardiovascular disease have both been related to a diet high in unhealthy fats such as fatty meats, butter, and fried meals.

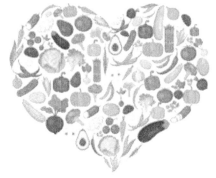

Sodium:

This mineral contributes to high blood pressure, particularly an increased risk of heart disease, and it is commonly found in processed foods, fast food, and restaurant meals.

The Heart-Healthy Cookbook is designed to help you make informed and delicious choices about what you eat. A compilation of delectable dishes that are healthy for your heart and taste buds can be found in this book. From breakfast to dinner and even desserts, you'll find a wide range of quick, easy meals packed with nutrients that are excellent for your heart. This cookbook includes information for everyone, regardless of whether their goal is to reduce weight, control their blood pressure, or maintain a healthy lifestyle.

This cookbook is an enjoyable and practical approach to start eating better and lowering your risk of cardiovascular disease. I understand that making significant dietary changes can be daunting, so I've designed the recipes to be simple, straightforward, and easy to follow.

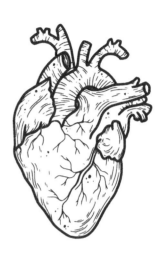

Each recipe in the cookbook has whole, nutrient-dense ingredients low in saturated and trans fats, sodium, and cholesterol. To ensure you get all the essential nutrients your body requires to thrive, we've included a range of vegetables, lean protein sources, fruits, whole grains, and healthy fats like nuts and seeds.

The cookbook gives helpful guidance on improving one's diet and leading a heart-healthy lifestyle in addition to tasty meals.

This cookbook is appropriate for all levels of cooks, experienced or novice. You may easily modify the recipes to fit your likes and preferences because they are versatile and adaptable.

FOOD TO AVOID

However, certain foods should be avoided or limited to maintain a healthy heart. We'll discuss the top foods to avoid for a heart-healthy diet and why they harm heart health.

Processed and Packaged Foods

Processed and packaged foods are often high in sodium, added sugars, and unhealthy fats. Salt contains sodium, which maintains the body's fluid equilibrium. A high salt diet, however, can raise blood pressure and strain the heart. The increased risk of obesity and cardiovascular disease is exacerbated by adding sugar and harmful fats to many processed and packaged foods. Limiting processed and sealed foods and opting for fresh, whole foods whenever possible is best for maintaining a heart-healthy diet.

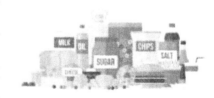

Red Meat

Red meat has a lot of saturated fat, raising cholesterol and the chance of developing heart disease. Furthermore, prepared meats like sausage, bacon, and deli meats are frequently rich in sodium and preservatives, which can harm cardiovascular health. Lean protein sources, including poultry, fish, beans, and lentils, are preferred over red meat to lower heart disease risk.

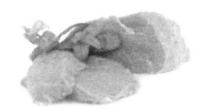

Fried Foods

Fried chicken, French fries, and fried fish are just a few examples of fried foods heavy in unhealthy fats and calories. Consuming too much fried food can increase cholesterol levels and contribute to weight gain, both risk factors for heart illness. To maintain a diet healthy for the heart, limiting fried food consumption and choosing more nutritional cooking methods like baking, broiling, or grilling is best.

Sugary Drinks

Sugary beverages with a lot of added sugar and calories include soda, sports, and energy drinks. Overindulging in sugar can cause weight gain and raise your chance of developing heart disease. Limiting the intake of sugary drinks and opting for healthier options like water, unsweetened tea, or sparkling water are the best ways to maintain a heart-healthy diet.

Processed Snacks

Chips, crackers, as well as cookies are just some examples of processed snacks that tend to be rich in sodium, added sugars, and unhealthy fats. Consuming unhealthy processed snacks has been linked to weight gain and an increased risk of cardiovascular disease. Limiting processed snack consumption and choosing healthier options like fresh fruit, vegetables, or nuts is best for maintaining a heart-healthy diet.

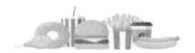

Butter and Margarine

Saturated and Trans fatty acids, found in abundance in butter and margarine, have been linked to elevated cholesterol as well as an increased risk of heart ailments. To maintain a heart-healthy diet, it is best to limit or avoid butter and margarine consumption and choose healthier options like olive oil, avocado, or nuts.

High-Fat Dairy Products

Cheese, as well as whole milk, are examples of high-fat dairy products that are also high in calories as well as saturated fat. Cholesterol and weight gain are risk factors for cardiovascular disease, and consuming excessive high-fat dairy can exacerbate both. Reduce your intake of full-fat dairy products and replace them with skim milk, low-fat cheese, or Greek yoghurt to keep your heart healthy.

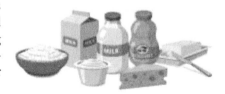

Baked Goods

Baked goods like cakes, cookies, and pastries are often high in added sugars and unhealthy fats. Overindulging in baked goods has been linked to weight gain and cardiovascular disease risk. Limiting baked goods consumption and choosing healthier options is best for maintaining a heart-healthy diet.

Maintaining a healthy cardiovascular system requires eating a heart-friendly diet. A heart-healthy diet comprises foods containing high minerals, fibre, as well as good fats while having low saturated and trans fats, cholesterol, and sodium.

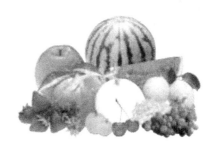

Veggies and fruits

Because of their high vitamin, mineral material, and fiber content, fruits and vegetables are essential to a diet that supports cardiovascular health. Calories aren't the only thing prevalent in these foods; antioxidants, which help reduce inflammation and protect the heart, are, too. Eat colourful produce dailies, such as berries, citrus fruits, leafy greens, and cruciferous veggies.

Whole Grains

Oatmeal, wheat bread, and other whole grain products are some of the best dietary sources of fibre, vitamins, and minerals. Whole grains reduce cholesterol and lower heart disease risk, but refined grains like those found in white pasta and bread elevate cholesterol and increase the risk of heart disease. Whole grains are an excellent option for weight management because they are filling.

Lean Protein Sources

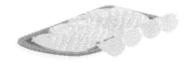

Poultry, fish, beans, and lentils are all examples of lean protein sources that are great for a heart-healthy diet since they are high in nutrients and saturated fats. Omega-3 fatty acids, found in abundance in fish, have been shown to reduce inflammation and the possibility of cardiovascular disease. Fish like salmon, mackerel, and tuna should comprise at least two weekly servings.

Seeds and Nuts

Seeds and nuts are excellent healthy fats, protein, and fibre sources. Eating nuts and seeds regularly can help reduce inflammation and decrease cholesterol levels, reducing the danger of heart ailments. A heart-healthy diet should include flaxseeds, chia seeds, almonds, and walnuts.

Healthy Fats

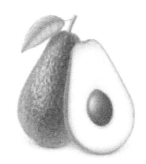

Monounsaturated and polyunsaturated fats, for example, are healthy fats that are good for the heart. The risk of heart disease can be decreased by these fats' ability to cut cholesterol levels and reduce inflammation. Nuts, avocados, and olive oil are all excellent sources of good fats.

Lactose-Free Dairy Products

Greek yoghurt, low-fat cheese, and skim milk are good providers of protein, calcium, and other necessary elements. Choosing low-fat dairy products over high-fat options can help reduce cholesterol levels and heart disease risk.

Herbs and Spices

You may flavor food with herbs and spices without excessive salt or bad fats. Garlic, ginger, turmeric, and cinnamons are some herbs and spices that can help lower cholesterol and inflammation, which reduces the risk of heart disease.

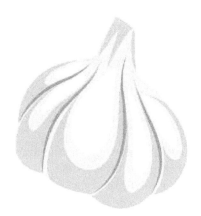

Chocolate, dark

The antioxidants known as flavonoids, abundant in dark chocolate, can help lower blood pressure and inflammation, decreasing the danger of heart problems. A heart-healthy diet can include a small amount of dark chocolate (at least 70% cocoa) daily.

Green Tea

Green tea has many catechins and antioxidants that can lower cholesterol and inflammation, reducing the risk of heart disease. Regularly drinking green tea can help you maintain a heart-healthy diet.

Water

Being hydrated is crucial for heart health and is necessary for general wellness. Water consumption throughout the day can help control blood pressure and lower the chance of developing heart disease.

BENEFITS OF HEART HEALTHY DIETS

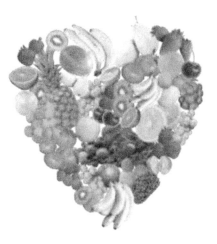

Eating a heart-healthy diet is crucial in reducing the danger of heart problems. Foods rich in saturated, as well as trans fats, sodium, and cholesterol, should be avoided, while those rich in fibre, minerals, and heart-healthy fats should be emphasized. In this article, we'll discuss the top benefits of a heart-healthy diet and why it is essential to maintain a healthy heart.

Reduces the Risk of Heart Disease

A healthy diet for the heart lowers the risk of developing heart disease, which is its main advantage. The blood arteries that feed the heart with oxygen and nutrients narrow or get blocked due to plaque formation, the world's leading cause of mortality. Consuming a diet low in fats that are saturated and trans, sodium, and cholesterol, yet high in mineral content, fibre, and healthy fats, can reduce your risk of developing heart problems.

Lowers Blood Pressure

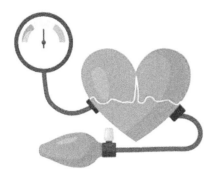

Heart disease is significantly increased by high blood pressure, frequently brought on by excess sodium intake. Consuming a heart-healthy diet that is rich in potassium as well as inadequate in sodium can help reduce blood pressure and the risk of developing heart problems.

Maintains Healthy Cholesterol Levels

Your blood contains a waxy material called cholesterol, and having high LDL cholesterol, or "bad" cholesterol, can raise your chance of getting heart disease. A diet that promotes cardiovascular is one that is low in trans fats and saturated fats and high in fibre and healthy fats, as well as may help you keep healthy cholesterol levels and reduce your chances of cardiovascular illness.

Encourages a Healthy Weight

Maintaining a healthy weight is vital to improving overall health and lowering the risk of heart disease. A high-fibre, low-calorie diet is associated with fewer health risks and better weight loss.

Reduces Inflammation

Although inflammation is a typical reaction to injury or illness, it can also be chronic, leading to heart disease. A heart-healthy diet full of anti-inflammatory and antioxidant-rich foods, such as fatty fish, whole grains, nuts, and veggies, can reduce inflammation and lower your risk of developing heart disease.

Improves Blood Sugar Control

Controlling the average level of blood sugar is essential for good health and can significantly reduce the chance of developing cardiovascular disease. Eating a diet rich in heart-healthy nutrients and fibre and relatively low in sugar will help you balance your blood sugar and reduce your risk of developing a cardiac disease.

Increases Energy and Improves Mood

Eating a diet that is good for the heart and high in nutrients and fats can give you more energy and make you feel better overall. Nutrient-dense foods provide your body with the vitamins, minerals, and antioxidants it needs to function correctly, while healthy fats help support brain function and mood regulation.

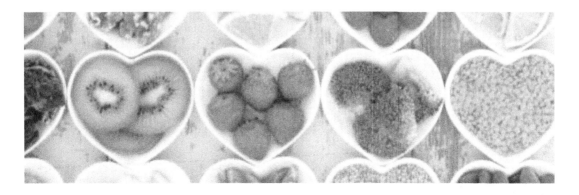

BEANS, GRAINS AND PASTA

Small Pasta and Beans Pot

Preparation time: 15 minutes

Cooking time: 15 minutes

Servings: 2-4

Ingredients:

- 1 pound (454 g) small whole wheat pasta
- 1 (14.5-ounce/411-g) can diced tomatoes, juice reserved
- 1 (15-ounce/425-g) can cannellini beans, drained and rinsed
- 2 tablespoons no-salt-added tomato paste
- 1 red or yellow bell pepper, chopped
- 1 yellow onion, chopped
- 1 tablespoon Italian seasoning mix
- 3 garlic cloves, minced
- ¼ teaspoon crushed red pepper flakes, optional
- 1 tablespoon extra-virgin olive oil
- 5 cups water
- 1 bunch kale, stemmed and chopped
- ½ cup pitted Klamath olives, chopped
- 1 cup sliced basil

Directions:

1. Except for the kale, olives, and basil, combine all the ingredients in a pot. Stir to mix well. Bring to a boil over high heat. Stir constantly.
2. Reduce the heat to medium high and add the kale. Cook for 10 minutes or until the pasta is al dente. Stir constantly. Transfer all of them on a large plate and serve with olives and basil on top.

Nutrition:

- ✓ Calories: 357
- ✓ Fat: 7.6g
- ✓ Protein: 18.2g
- ✓ Carbs: 64.5g

Wild Rice, Celery, and Cauliflower Pilaf

Preparation time: 15 minutes

Cooking time: 45 minutes

Servings: 4

Ingredients:

- 1 tablespoon olive oil, plus more for greasing the baking dish
- 1 cup wild rice
- 2 cups low-sodium chicken broth
- 1 sweet onion, chopped
- 2 stalks celery, chopped
- 1 teaspoon minced garlic
- 2 carrots, peeled, halved lengthwise, and sliced
- ½ cauliflower head, cut into small florets
- 1 teaspoon chopped fresh thyme
- Sea salt, to taste

Directions:

1. Preheat the oven to 350°f (180°c). Line a baking sheet with parchment paper and grease with olive oil.
2. Put the wild rice in a saucepan, then pour in the chicken broth. Bring to a boil. Reduce the heat to low and simmer for 30 minutes or until the rice is plump.
3. Meanwhile, heat the remaining olive oil in an oven-proof skillet over medium-high heat until shimmering.
4. Add the onion, celery, and garlic to the skillet and sauté for 3 minutes or until the onion is translucent.
5. Add the carrots and cauliflower to the skillet and sauté for 5 minutes. Turn off the heat and set aside.
6. Pour the cooked rice in the skillet with the vegetables. Sprinkle with thyme and salt. Set the skillet in the preheated oven and bake for 15 minutes or until the vegetables are soft. Serve immediately.

Nutrition:

- ✓ Calories: 214
- ✓ Fat: 3.9g
- ✓ Protein: 7.2g

✓ Carbs: 37.9g

Minestrone Chickpeas and Macaroni Casserole

Preparation time: 15 minutes

Cooking time: 7 hours & 25 minutes

Servings: 5

Ingredients:

- 1 (15-ounce/425-g) can chickpeas, drained and rinsed
- 1 (28-ounce/794-g) can diced tomatoes, with the juice
- 1 (6-ounce/170-g) can no-salt-added tomato paste
- 3 medium carrots, sliced
- 3 cloves garlic, minced
- 1 medium yellow onion, chopped
- 1 cup low-sodium vegetable soup
- ½ teaspoon dried rosemary
- 1 teaspoon dried oregano
- 2 teaspoons maple syrup
- ½ teaspoon sea salt
- ¼ teaspoon ground black pepper
- ½ pound (227-g) fresh green beans, trimmed and cut into bite-size pieces
- 1 cup macaroni pasta
- 2 ounces (57 g) Parmesan cheese, grated

Directions:

1. Except for the green beans, pasta, and Parmesan cheese, combine all the ingredients in the slow cooker and stir to mix well. Put the slow cooker lid on and cook on low for 7 hours.
2. Fold in the pasta and green beans. Put the lid on and cook on high for 20 minutes or until the vegetable are soft and the pasta is al dente.
3. Pour them in a large serving bowl and spread with Parmesan cheese before serving.

Nutrition:

- ✓ Calories: 349
- ✓ Fat: 6.7g
- ✓ Protein: 16.5g

✓ Carbs: 59.9g

Slow Cooked Turkey and Brown Rice

Preparation time: 15 minutes

Cooking time: 3 hours & 10 minutes

Servings: 6

Ingredients:

- 1 tablespoon extra-virgin olive oil
- 1½ pounds (680 g) ground turkey
- 2 tablespoons chopped fresh sage, divided
- 2 tablespoons chopped fresh thyme, divided
- 1 teaspoon sea salt
- ½ teaspoon ground black pepper
- 2 cups brown rice
- 1 (14-ounce / 397-g) can stewed tomatoes, with the juice
- ¼ cup pitted and sliced Klamath olives
- 3 medium zucchinis, sliced thinly
- ¼ cup chopped fresh flat-leaf parsley
- 1 medium yellow onion, chopped
- 1 tablespoon plus 1 teaspoon balsamic vinegar
- 2 cups low-sodium chicken stock
- 2 garlic cloves, minced
- ½ cup grated Parmesan cheese, for serving

Directions:

1. Heat the olive oil in a nonstick skillet over medium-high heat until shimmering. Add the ground turkey and sprinkle with 1 tablespoon of sage, 1 tablespoon of thyme, salt and ground black pepper.
2. Sauté for 10 minutes or until the ground turkey is lightly browned. Pour them in the slow cooker, then pour in the remaining ingredients, except for the Parmesan. Stir to mix well.
3. Put the lid on and cook on high for 3 hours or until the rice and vegetables are tender. Pour them in a large serving bowl, then spread with Parmesan cheese before serving.

Nutrition:

- ✓ Calories: 499
- ✓ Fat: 16.4g
- ✓ Protein: 32.4g
- ✓ Carbs: 56.5g

Papaya, Jicama, and Peas Rice Bowl

Preparation time: 15 minutes

Cooking time: 45 minutes

Servings: 4

Ingredients:

Sauce:

- Juice of ¼ lemon
- 2 teaspoons chopped fresh basil
- 1 tablespoon raw honey
- 1 tablespoon extra-virgin olive oil
- Sea salt, to taste

Rice:

- 1½ cups wild rice
- 2 papayas, peeled, seeded, and diced
- 1 jicama, peeled and shredded
- 1 cup snow peas, julienned
- 2 cups shredded cabbage
- 1 scallion, white and green parts, chopped

Directions:

1. Combine the ingredients for the sauce in a bowl. Stir to mix well. Set aside until ready to use. Pour the wild rice in a saucepan, then pour in enough water to cover. Bring to a boil.
2. Reduce the heat to low, then simmer for 45 minutes or until the wild rice is soft and plump. Drain and transfer to a large serving bowl.
3. Top the rice with papayas, jicama, peas, cabbage, and scallion. Pour the sauce over and stir to mix well before serving.

Nutrition:

- ✓ Calories: 446
- ✓ Fat: 7.9g
- ✓ Protein: 13.1g
- ✓ Carbs: 85.8g

Italian Baked Beans

Preparation time: 5 minutes

Cooking time: 15 minutes

Servings: 6

Ingredients:

- 2 teaspoons extra-virgin olive oil
- ½ cup minced onion (about ¼ onion)
- 1 (12-ounce) can low-sodium tomato paste
- ¼ cup red wine vinegar
- 2 tablespoons honey
- ¼ teaspoon ground cinnamon
- ½ cup water
- 2 (15-ounce) cans cannellini or great northern beans, undrained

Directions:

1. In a medium saucepan over medium heat, heat the oil. Add the onion and cook for 5 minutes, stirring frequently.
2. Add the tomato paste, vinegar, honey, cinnamon, and water, and mix well. Turn the heat to low. Drain and rinse one can of the beans in a colander and add to the saucepan.
3. Pour the entire second can of beans (including the liquid) into the saucepan. Let it cook for 10 minutes, stirring occasionally, and serve.
4. Ingredient tip: Switch up this recipe by making new variations of the homemade ketchup. Instead of the cinnamon, try ¼ teaspoon of smoked paprika and 1 tablespoon of hot sauce. Serve.

Nutrition:

- ✓ Calories: 236
- ✓ Fat: 3g
- ✓ Carbohydrates: 42g
- ✓ Protein: 10g

Cannellini Bean Lettuce Wraps

Preparation time: 15 minutes

Cooking time: 10 minutes

Servings: 4

Ingredients:

- 1 tablespoon extra-virgin olive oil
- ½ cup diced red onion (about ¼ onion)
- ¾ cup chopped fresh tomatoes (about 1 medium tomato)
- ¼ teaspoon freshly ground black pepper
- 1 (15-ounce) can cannellini or great northern beans, drained and rinsed
- ¼ cup finely chopped fresh curly parsley
- ½ cup Lemony Garlic Hummus or ½ cup prepared hummus
- 8 romaine lettuce leaves

Directions:

1. In a large skillet over medium heat, heat the oil. Add the onion and cook for 3 minutes, stirring occasionally.
2. Add the tomatoes and pepper and cook for 3 more minutes, stirring occasionally. Add the beans and cook for 3 more minutes, stirring occasionally. Remove from the heat, and mix in the parsley.
3. Spread 1 tablespoon of hummus over each lettuce leaf. Evenly spread the warm bean mixture down the center of each leaf.
4. Fold one side of the lettuce leaf over the filling lengthwise, then fold over the other side to make a wrap and serve.

Nutrition:

- ✓ Calories: 211
- ✓ Fat: 8g
- ✓ Carbohydrates: 28g
- ✓ Protein: 10g

Israeli Eggplant, Chickpea, and Mint Sauté

Preparation time: 5 minutes

Cooking time: 20 minutes

Servings: 6

Ingredients:

- Nonstick cooking spray
- 1 medium globe eggplant (about 1 pound), stem removed
- 1 tablespoon extra-virgin olive oil
- 2 tablespoons freshly squeezed lemon juice (from about 1 small lemon)
- 2 tablespoons balsamic vinegar
- 1 teaspoon ground cumin
- ¼ teaspoon kosher or sea salt
- 1 (15-ounce) can chickpeas, drained and rinsed
- 1 cup sliced sweet onion (about ½ medium Walla Walla or Vidalia onion)
- ¼ cup loosely packed chopped or torn mint leaves
- 1 tablespoon sesame seeds, toasted if desired
- 1 garlic clove, finely minced (about ½ teaspoon)

Directions:

1. Place one oven rack about 4 inches below the broiler element. Turn the broiler to the highest setting to preheat. Spray a large, rimmed baking sheet with nonstick cooking spray.
2. On a cutting board, cut the eggplant lengthwise into four slabs (each piece should be about ½- to 1/8-inch thick). Place the eggplant slabs on the prepared baking sheet. Set aside.
3. In a small bowl, whisk together the oil, lemon juice, vinegar, cumin, and salt. Brush or drizzle 2 tablespoons of the lemon dressing over both sides of the eggplant slabs. Reserve the remaining dressing.
4. Broil the eggplant directly under the heating element for 4 minutes, flip them, and then broil for another 4 minutes, until golden brown.
5. While the eggplant is broiling, in a serving bowl, combine the chickpeas, onion, mint, sesame seeds, and garlic. Add the reserved dressing, and gently mix to incorporate all the ingredients.
6. When the eggplant is done, using tongs, transfer the slabs from the baking sheet to a cooling rack and cool for 3 minutes.
7. When slightly cooled, place the eggplant on a cutting board and slice each slab crosswise into ½-inch strips.
8. Add the eggplant to the serving bowl with the onion mixture. Gently toss everything together and serve warm or at room temperature.

- ✓ Calories: 159
- ✓ Fat: 4g
- ✓ Carbohydrates: 26g
- ✓ Protein: 6g

Lentils and Rice

Preparation time: 5 minutes

Cooking time: 25 minutes

Servings: 4

Ingredients:

- 2¼ cups low-sodium or no-salt-added vegetable broth
- ½ cup uncooked brown or green lentils
- ½ cup uncooked instant brown rice
- ½ cup diced carrots (about 1 carrot)
- ½ cup diced celery (about 1 stalk)
- 1 (2.25-ounce) can sliced olives, drained (about ½ cup)
- ¼ cup diced red onion (about 1/8 onion)
- ¼ cup chopped fresh curly-leaf parsley
- 1½ tablespoons extra-virgin olive oil
- 1 tablespoon freshly squeezed lemon juice (from about ½ small lemon)
- 1 garlic clove, minced (about ½ teaspoon)
- ¼ teaspoon kosher or sea salt
- ¼ teaspoon freshly ground black pepper

Directions:

1. In a medium saucepan over high heat, bring the broth and lentils to a boil, cover, and lower the heat to medium-low. Cook for 8 minutes.
2. Raise the heat to medium and stir in the rice. Cover the pot and cook the mixture for 15 minutes, or until the liquid is absorbed. Remove the pot from the heat and let it sit, covered, for 1 minute, then stir.
3. While the lentils and rice are cooking, mix together the carrots, celery, olives, onion, and parsley in a large serving bowl.
4. In a small bowl, whisk together the oil, lemon juice, garlic, salt, and pepper. Set aside. When the lentils and rice are cooked, add them to the serving bowl.

5. Pour the dressing on top and mix everything together. Serve warm or cold, or store in a sealed container in the refrigerator for up to 7 days.

Nutrition:

- ✓ Calories: 230
- ✓ Fat: 8g
- ✓ Carbohydrates: 34g
- ✓ Protein: 8g

Brown Rice Pilaf with Pistachios and Raisins

Preparation time: 15 minutes

Cooking time: 15 minutes

Servings: 6

Ingredients:

- 1 tablespoon extra-virgin olive oil
- 1 cup chopped onion
- ½ cup shredded carrot
- ½ teaspoon ground cinnamon
- 1 teaspoon ground cumin
- 2 cups brown rice
- 1¾ cups pure orange juice
- ¼ cup water
- ½ cup shelled pistachios
- 1 cup golden raisins
- ½ cup chopped fresh chives

Directions:

1. Heat the olive oil in a saucepan over medium-high heat until shimmering. Add the onion and sauté for 5 minutes or until translucent.
2. Add the carrots, cinnamon, and cumin, then sauté for 1 minutes or until aromatic.
3. Pour into the brown rice, orange juice, and water. Bring to a boil. Reduce the heat to medium-low and simmer for 7 minutes or until the liquid is almost absorbed.
4. Transfer the rice mixture in a large serving bowl, then spread with pistachios, raisins, and chives. Serve immediately.

Nutrition:

- ✓ Calories: 264

- ✓ Fat: 7.1g
- ✓ Protein: 5.2g
- ✓ Carbs: 48.9g

Cherry, Apricot, and Pecan Brown Rice Bowl

Preparation time: 15 minutes

Cooking time: 1 hour & 1 minute

Servings: 2

Ingredients:

- 2 tablespoons olive oil
- 2 green onions, sliced
- ½ cup brown rice
- 1 cup low -sodium chicken stock
- 2 tablespoons dried cherries
- 4 dried apricots, chopped
- 2 tablespoons pecans, toasted and chopped
- Sea salt and freshly ground pepper, to taste

Directions:

1. Heat the olive oil in a medium saucepan over medium-high heat until shimmering. Add the green onions and sauté for 1 minutes or until fragrant.
2. Add the rice. Stir to mix well, then pour in the chicken stock. Bring to a boil. Reduce the heat to low. Cover and simmer for 50 minutes or until the brown rice is soft.
3. Add the cherries, apricots, and pecans, and simmer for 10 more minutes or until the fruits are tender.
4. Pour them in a large serving bowl. Fluff with a fork. Sprinkle with sea salt and freshly ground pepper. Serve immediately.

Nutrition:

- ✓ Calories: 451
- ✓ Fat: 25.9g
- ✓ Protein: 8.2g
- ✓ Carbs: 50.4g

Curry Apple Couscous with Leeks and Pecans

Preparation time: 15 minutes

Cooking time: 8 minutes

Servings: 4

Ingredients:

- 2 teaspoons extra-virgin olive oil
- 2 leeks, white parts only, sliced
- 1 apple, diced
- 2 cups cooked couscous
- 2 tablespoons curry powder
- ½ cup chopped pecans

Directions:

1. Heat the olive oil in a skillet over medium heat until shimmering. Add the leeks and sauté for 5 minutes or until soft.
2. Add the diced apple and cook for 3 more minutes until tender. Add the couscous and curry powder. Stir to combine. Transfer them in a large serving bowl, then mix in the pecans and serve.

Nutrition:

- ✓ Calories: 254
- ✓ Fat: 11.9g
- ✓ Protein: 5.4g
- ✓ Carbs: 34.3g

Lebanese Flavor Broken Thin Noodles

Preparation time: 15 minutes

Cooking time: 25 minutes

Servings: 6

Ingredients:

- 1 tablespoon extra-virgin olive oil
- 1 (3-ounce / 85-g) cup vermicelli, broken into 1- to 1½-inch pieces
- 3 cups shredded cabbage
- 1 cup brown rice
- 3 cups low-sodium vegetable soup
- ½ cup water
- 2 garlic cloves, mashed
- ¼ teaspoon sea salt
- 1/8 teaspoon crushed red pepper flakes
- ½ cup coarsely chopped cilantro
- Fresh lemon slices, for serving

Directions:

1. Heat the olive oil in a saucepan over medium-high heat until shimmering. Add the vermicelli and sauté for 3 minutes or until toasted. Add the cabbage and sauté for 4 minutes or until tender.
2. Pour in the brown rice, vegetable soup, and water. Add the garlic and sprinkle with salt and red pepper flakes.
3. Bring to a boil over high heat. Reduce the heat to medium low. Put the lid on and simmer for another 10 minutes. Turn off the heat, then let sit for 5 minutes without opening the lid.
4. Pour them on a large serving platter and spread with cilantro. Squeeze the lemon slices over and serve warm.

Nutrition:

- ✓ Calories: 127
- ✓ Fat: 3.1g
- ✓ Protein: 4.2g
- ✓ Carbs: 22.9g

Lemony Farro and Avocado Bowl

Preparation time: 15 minutes

Cooking time: 25 minutes

Servings: 4

Ingredients:

- 1 tablespoon plus 2 teaspoons extra-virgin olive oil, divided
- ½ medium onion, chopped
- 1 carrot, shredded
- 2 garlic cloves, minced
- 1 (6-ounce / 170-g) cup pearled farro
- 2 cups low-sodium vegetable soup
- 2 avocados, peeled, pitted, and sliced
- Zest and juice of 1 small lemon
- ¼ teaspoon sea salt

Directions:

1. Heat 1 tablespoon of olive oil in a saucepan over medium-high heat until shimmering. Add the onion and sauté for 5 minutes or until translucent. Add the carrot and garlic and sauté for 1 minute or until fragrant.

2. Add the farro and pour in the vegetable soup. Bring to a boil over high heat. Reduce the heat to low. Put the lid on and simmer for 20 minutes or until the farro is al dente.
3. Transfer the farro in a large serving bowl, then fold in the avocado slices. Sprinkle with lemon zest and salt, then drizzle with lemon juice and 2 teaspoons of olive oil. Stir to mix well and serve immediately.

Nutrition:

- ✓ Calories: 210
- ✓ Fat: 11.1g
- ✓ Protein: 4.2g
- ✓ Carbs: 27.9g

Rice and Blueberry Stuffed Sweet Potatoes

Preparation time: 15 minutes

Cooking time: 20 minutes

Servings: 4

Ingredients:

- 2 cups cooked wild rice
- ½ cup dried blueberries
- ½ cup chopped hazelnuts
- ½ cup shredded Swiss chard
- 1 teaspoon chopped fresh thyme
- 1 scallion, white and green parts, peeled and thinly sliced
- Sea salt and freshly ground black pepper, to taste
- 4 sweet potatoes, baked in the skin until tender

Directions:

1. Preheat the oven to 400°f (205°c). Combine all the ingredients, except for the sweet potatoes, in a large bowl. Stir to mix well.
2. Cut the top third of the sweet potato off length wire, then scoop most of the sweet potato flesh out. Fill the potato with the wild rice mixture, then set the sweet potato on a greased baking sheet.

3. Bake in the preheated oven for 20 minutes or until the sweet potato skin is lightly charred. Serve immediately.

Nutrition:

- ✓ Calories: 393
- ✓ Fat: 7.1g
- ✓ Protein: 10.2g
- ✓ Carbs: 76.9g

Farrotto Mix

Preparation time: 15 minutes

Cooking time: 40 minutes

Servings: 6

Ingredients:

- ½ onion, chopped fine
- 1 cup frozen peas, thawed
- 1 garlic clove, minced
- 1 tablespoon minced fresh chives
- 1 teaspoon grated lemon zest plus 1 teaspoon juice
- 1½ cups whole farro
- 1½ ounces Parmesan cheese, grated (¾ cup)
- 2 tablespoons extra-virgin olive oil
- 2 teaspoons minced fresh tarragon
- 3 cups chicken broth
- 3 cups water
- 4 ounces asparagus, trimmed and cut on bias into 1-inch lengths
- 4 ounces pancetta, cut into ¼-inch pieces
- Salt and pepper

Directions:

1. Pulse farro using a blender until about half of grains are broken into smaller pieces, about 6 pulses.
2. Bring broth and water to boil in moderate-sized saucepan on high heat. Put in asparagus and cook until crisp-tender, 2 to 3 minutes.
3. Use a slotted spoon to move asparagus to a container and set aside. Decrease heat to low, cover broth mixture, and keep warm.

4. Cook pancetta in a Dutch oven on moderate heat until lightly browned and fat has rendered, approximately 5 minutes.
5. Put in 1 tablespoon oil and onion and cook till they become tender, approximately 5 minutes. Mix in garlic and cook until aromatic, approximately half a minute.
6. Put in farro and cook, stirring often, until grains are lightly toasted, approximately three minutes.
7. Stir 5 cups warm broth mixture into farro mixture, decrease the heat to low, cover, and cook until almost all liquid has been absorbed and farro is just al dente, about 25 minutes, stirring twice during cooking.
8. Put in peas, tarragon, ¾ teaspoon salt, and ½ teaspoon pepper and cook, stirring continuously, until farro becomes creamy, approximately 5 minutes.
9. Remove from the heat, mix in Parmesan, chives, lemon zest and juice, remaining 1 tablespoon oil, and reserved asparagus.
10. Adjust consistency with remaining warm broth mixture as required (you may have broth left over). Sprinkle with salt and pepper to taste. Serve.

Nutrition:

- ✓ Calories: 218
- ✓ Carbs: 41g
- ✓ Fat: 2g
- ✓ Protein: 7g

Feta-Grape-Bulgur Salad with Grapes and Feta

Preparation time: 15 minutes

Cooking time: 1 hour & 30 minutes

Servings: 4-6

Ingredients:

- ¼ cup chopped fresh mint
- ¼ cup extra-virgin olive oil
- ¼ teaspoon ground cumin
- ½ cup slivered almonds, toasted
- 1 cup water
- 1½ cups medium-grind bulgur, rinsed
- 2 ounces feta cheese, crumbled (½ cup)
- 2 scallions, sliced thin

- 5 tablespoons lemon juice (2 lemons)
- 6 ounces seedless red grapes, quartered (1 cup)
- Pinch cayenne pepper
- Salt and pepper

Directions:

1. Mix bulgur, water, ¼ cup lemon juice, and ¼ teaspoon salt in a container. Cover and allow to sit at room temperature until grains are softened and liquid is fully absorbed, about 1½ hours.
2. Beat remaining 1 tablespoon lemon juice, oil, cumin, cayenne, and ¼ teaspoon salt together in a big container.
3. Put in bulgur, grapes, 1/3 cup almonds, 1/3 cup feta, scallions, and mint and gently toss to combine. Sprinkle with salt and pepper to taste. Sprinkle with remaining almonds and remaining feta before you serve.

Nutrition:

- ✓ Calories: 500
- ✓ Carbs: 45g
- ✓ Fat: 14g
- ✓ Protein: 50g

Greek Style Meaty Bulgur

Preparation time: 15 minutes

Cooking time: 30 minutes

Servings: 4-6

Ingredients:

- ½ cup jarred roasted red peppers, rinsed, patted dry, and chopped
- 1 bay leaf
- 1 cup medium-grind bulgur, rinsed
- 1 onion, chopped fine
- 1 tablespoon chopped fresh dill
- 1 teaspoon extra-virgin olive oil
- 1 1/3 cups vegetable broth
- 2 teaspoons minced fresh marjoram or ½ teaspoon dried
- 3 garlic cloves, minced
- 8 ounces ground lamb

- Lemon wedges
- Salt and pepper

Directions:

1. Heat oil in a big saucepan on moderate to high heat until just smoking. Put in lamb, ½ teaspoon salt, and ¼ teaspoon pepper and cook, breaking up meat with wooden spoon, until browned, 3 to 5 minutes.
2. Mix in onion and red peppers and cook until onion is softened, 5 to 7 minutes. Mix in garlic and marjoram and cook until aromatic, approximately half a minute.
3. Mix in bulgur, broth, and bay leaf and bring to simmer. Decrease heat to low, cover, and simmer gently until bulgur is tender, 16 to 18 minutes.
4. Remove from the heat, lay clean dish towel underneath lid and let bulgur sit for about 10 minutes.
5. Put in dill and fluff gently with fork to combine. Sprinkle with salt and pepper to taste. Serve with lemon wedges.

Nutrition:

- ✓ Calories: 137
- ✓ Carbs: 16g
- ✓ Fat: 5g
- ✓ Protein: 7g

Hearty Barley Mix

Preparation time: 15 minutes

Cooking time: 50 minutes

Servings: 4

Ingredients:

- 1/8 teaspoon ground cardamom
- ½ cup plain yogurt
- ½ teaspoon ground cumin
- 2/3 cup raw sunflower seeds
- ¾ teaspoon ground coriander
- 1 cup pearl barley
- 1½ tablespoons minced fresh mint
- 1½ teaspoons grated lemon zest plus 1½ tablespoons juice
- 3 tablespoons extra-virgin olive oil
- 5 carrots, peeled

- 8 ounces snow peas, strings removed, halved along the length
- Salt and pepper

Directions:

1. Beat yogurt, ½ teaspoon lemon zest and 1½ teaspoons juice, 1½ teaspoons mint, ¼ teaspoon salt, and 1/8 teaspoon pepper together in a small-sized container; cover put inside your fridge until ready to serve.
2. Bring 4 quarts water to boil in a Dutch oven. Put in barley and 1 tablespoon salt, return to boil, and cook until tender, 20 to 40 minutes. Drain barley, return to now-empty pot, and cover to keep warm.
3. In the meantime, halve carrots crosswise, then halve or quarter along the length to create uniformly sized pieces.
4. Heat 1 tablespoon oil in 12-inch frying pan on moderate to high heat until just smoking. Put in carrots and ½ teaspoon coriander and cook, stirring intermittently, until mildly charred and just tender, 5 to 7 minutes.
5. Put in snow peas and cook, stirring intermittently, until spotty brown, 3 to 5 minutes; move to plate.
6. Heat 1½ teaspoons oil in now-empty frying pan on moderate heat until it starts to shimmer. Put in sunflower seeds, cumin, cardamom, remaining ¼ teaspoon coriander, and ¼ teaspoon salt.
7. Cook, stirring continuously, until seeds are toasted, approximately 2 minutes; move to small-sized container.
8. Beat remaining 1 teaspoon lemon zest and 1 tablespoon juice, remaining 1 tablespoon mint, and remaining 1½ tablespoons oil together in a big container.
9. Put in barley and carrot–snow pea mixture and gently toss to combine. Sprinkle with salt and pepper to taste. Serve, topping individual portions with spiced sunflower seeds and drizzling with yogurt sauce.

Nutrition:

- ✓ Calories: 193
- ✓ Carbs: 44g
- ✓ Fat: 1g
- ✓ Protein: 4g

Hearty Barley Risotto

Preparation time: 15 minutes

Cooking time: 60 minutes

Servings: 4-6

Ingredients:

- 1 carrot, peeled and chopped fine
- 1 cup dry white wine
- 1 onion, chopped fine
- 1 teaspoon minced fresh thyme or ¼ teaspoon dried
- 1½ cups pearl barley
- 2 ounces Parmesan cheese, grated (1 cup)
- 2 tablespoons extra-virgin olive oil
- 4 cups chicken or vegetable broth
- 4 cups water
- Salt and pepper

Directions:

1. Bring broth and water to simmer in moderate-sized saucepan. Decrease heat to low and cover to keep warm.
2. Heat 1 tablespoon oil in a Dutch oven on moderate heat until it starts to shimmer. Put in onion and carrot and cook till they become tender, 5 to 7 minutes.
3. Put in barley and cook, stirring frequently, until lightly toasted and aromatic, about 4 minutes. Put in wine and cook, stirring often, until fully absorbed, approximately two minutes.
4. Mix in 3 cups warm broth and thyme, bring to simmer, and cook, stirring intermittently, until liquid is absorbed and bottom of pot is dry, 22 to 25 minutes.
5. Mix in 2 cups warm broth, bring to simmer, and cook, stirring intermittently, until liquid is absorbed and bottom of pot is dry, fifteen to twenty minutes.
6. Carry on cooking risotto, stirring frequently and adding warm broth as required to stop pot bottom from becoming dry, until barley is cooked through, 15 to 20 minutes.
7. Remove from the heat, adjust consistency with remaining warm broth as required. Mix in Parmesan and residual 1 tablespoon

oil and sprinkle with salt and pepper to taste. Serve.

Nutrition:

- ✓ Calories: 222
- ✓ Carbs: 33g
- ✓ Fat: 5g
- ✓ Protein: 6g

Hearty Freekeh Pilaf

Preparation time: 15 minutes

Cooking time: 60 minutes

Servings: 4-6

Ingredients:

- ¼ cup chopped fresh mint
- ¼ cup extra-virgin olive oil, plus extra for serving
- ¼ cup shelled pistachios, toasted and coarsely chopped
- ¼ teaspoon ground coriander
- ¼ teaspoon ground cumin
- 1 head cauliflower (2 pounds), cored and cut into ½-inch florets
- 1 shallot, minced
- 1½ cups whole freekeh
- 1½ tablespoons lemon juice
- 1½ teaspoons grated fresh ginger
- 3 ounces pitted dates, chopped (½ cup)
- Salt and pepper

Directions:

1. Bring 4 quarts water to boil in a Dutch oven. Put in freekeh and 1 tablespoon salt, return to boil, and cook until grains are tender, 30 to 45 minutes. Drain freekeh, return to now-empty pot, and cover to keep warm.
2. Heat 2 tablespoons oil in 12-inch non-stick frying pan on moderate to high heat until it starts to shimmer.
3. Put in cauliflower, ½ teaspoon salt, and ¼ teaspoon pepper, cover, and cook until florets are softened and start to brown, approximately five minutes.
4. Remove lid and continue to cook, stirring intermittently, until florets turn spotty brown, about 10 minutes.

5. Put in remaining 2 tablespoons oil, dates, shallot, ginger, coriander, and cumin and cook, stirring often, until dates and shallot are softened and aromatic, approximately 3 minutes.
6. Decrease heat to low, put in freekeh, and cook, stirring often, until heated through, about 1 minute. Remove from the heat, mix in pistachios, mint, and lemon juice.
7. Sprinkle with salt and pepper to taste and drizzle with extra oil. Serve.

Nutrition:

- ✓ Calories: 520
- ✓ Carbs: 54g
- ✓ Fat: 14g
- ✓ Protein: 36g

Herby-Lemony Farro

Preparation time: 15 minutes

Cooking time: 40 minutes

Servings: 4-6

Ingredients:

- ¼ cup chopped fresh mint
- ¼ cup chopped fresh parsley
- 1 garlic clove, minced
- 1 onion, chopped fine
- 1 tablespoon lemon juice
- 1½ cups whole farro
- 3 tablespoons extra-virgin olive oil
- Salt and pepper

Directions:

1. Bring 4 quarts water to boil in a Dutch oven. Put in farro and 1 tablespoon salt, return to boil, and cook until grains are soft with slight chew, 15 to 30 minutes. Drain farro, return to now-empty pot, and cover to keep warm.
2. Heat 2 tablespoons oil in 12-inch frying pan on moderate heat until it starts to shimmer. Put in onion and ¼ teaspoon salt and cook till they become tender, approximately five minutes.
3. Mix in garlic and cook until aromatic, approximately half a minute. Put in residual 1 tablespoon oil and farro and

cook, stirring often, until heated through, approximately two minutes.

4. Remove from the heat, mix in parsley, mint, and lemon juice. Sprinkle with salt and pepper to taste. Serve.

Nutrition:

- ✓ Calories: 243
- ✓ Carbs: 22g
- ✓ Fat: 14g
- ✓ Protein: 10g

Mushroom-Bulgur Pilaf

Preparation time: 15 minutes

Cooking time: 30 minutes

Servings: 4

Ingredients:

- ¼ cup minced fresh parsley
- ¼ ounce dried porcini mushrooms, rinsed and minced
- ¾ cup chicken or vegetable broth
- ¾ cup water
- 1 cup medium-grind bulgur, rinsed
- 1 onion, chopped fine
- 2 garlic cloves, minced
- 2 tablespoons extra-virgin olive oil
- 8 ounces cremini mushrooms, trimmed, halved if small or quartered if large
- Salt and pepper

Directions:

1. Heat oil in a big saucepan on moderate heat until it starts to shimmer. Put in onion, porcini mushrooms, and ½ teaspoon salt and cook until onion is softened, approximately 5 minutes.
2. Mix in cremini mushrooms, increase heat to medium-high, cover, and cook until cremini release their liquid and begin to brown, about 4 minutes.
3. Mix in garlic and cook until aromatic, approximately half a minute. Mix in bulgur, broth, and water and bring to simmer.
4. Decrease heat to low, cover, and simmer gently until bulgur is tender, 16 to 18 minutes. Remove from the heat, lay clean

dish towel underneath lid and let pilaf sit for about ten minutes.

5. Put in parsley to pilaf and fluff gently with fork to combine. Sprinkle with salt and pepper to taste. Serve.

Nutrition:

- ✓ Calories: 259
- ✓ Carbs: 50g
- ✓ Fat: 3g
- ✓ Protein: 11g

Baked Brown Rice

Preparation time: 15 minutes

Cooking time: 1 hour & 25 minutes

Servings: 4-6

Ingredients:

- ½ cup minced fresh parsley
- ¾ cup jarred roasted red peppers, rinsed, patted dry, and chopped
- 1 cup chicken or vegetable broth
- 1½ cups long-grain brown rice, rinsed
- 2 onions, chopped fine
- 2¼ cups water
- 4 teaspoons extra-virgin olive oil
- Grated Parmesan cheese
- Lemon wedges
- Salt and pepper

Directions:

1. Place the oven rack in the center of the oven and pre-heat your oven to 375 degrees. Heat oil in a Dutch oven on moderate heat until it starts to shimmer.
2. Put in onions and 1 teaspoon salt and cook, stirring intermittently, till they become tender and well browned, 12 to 14 minutes.
3. Mix in water and broth and bring to boil. Mix in rice, cover, and move pot to oven. Bake until rice becomes soft and liquid is absorbed, 65 to 70 minutes.
4. Remove pot from oven. Sprinkle red peppers over rice, cover, and allow to sit for about five minutes.
5. Put in parsley to rice and fluff gently with fork to combine. Sprinkle with salt and

pepper to taste. Serve with grated Parmesan and lemon wedges.

Nutrition:

- ✓ Calories: 100
- ✓ Carbs: 27g
- ✓ Fat: 21g
- ✓ Protein: 2g

Barley Pilaf

Preparation time: 15 minutes

Cooking time: 45 minutes

Servings: 4-6

Ingredients:

- ¼ cup minced fresh parsley
- 1 small onion, chopped fine
- 1½ cups pearl barley, rinsed
- 1½ teaspoons lemon juice
- 1½ teaspoons minced fresh thyme or ½ teaspoon dried
- 2 garlic cloves, minced
- 2 tablespoons minced fresh chives
- 2½ cups water
- 3 tablespoons extra-virgin olive oil
- Salt and pepper

Directions:

1. Heat oil in a big saucepan on moderate heat until it starts to shimmer. Put in onion and ½ teaspoon salt and cook till they become tender, approximately 5 minutes.
2. Mix in barley, garlic, and thyme and cook, stirring often, until barley is lightly toasted and aromatic, approximately three minutes.
3. Mix in water and bring to simmer. Decrease heat to low, cover, and simmer until barley becomes soft and water is absorbed, 20 to 40 minutes.
4. Remove from the heat, lay clean dish towel underneath lid and let pilaf sit for about ten minutes. Put in parsley, chives, and lemon juice to pilaf and fluff gently with fork to combine. Sprinkle with salt and pepper to taste. Serve.

Nutrition:

- ✓ Calories: 39
- ✓ Carbs: 8g
- ✓ Fat: 1g
- ✓ Protein: 1g

Basmati Rice Pilaf Mix

Preparation time: 15 minutes

Cooking time: 25 minutes

Servings: 4-6

Ingredients:

- ¼ cup currants
- ¼ cup sliced almonds, toasted
- ¼ teaspoon ground cinnamon
- ½ teaspoon ground turmeric
- 1 small onion, chopped fine
- 1 tablespoon extra-virgin olive oil
- 1½ cups basmati rice, rinsed
- 2 garlic cloves, minced
- 2¼ cups water
- Salt and pepper

Directions:

1. Heat oil in a big saucepan on moderate heat until it starts to shimmer. Put in onion and ¼ teaspoon salt and cook till they become tender, approximately 5 minutes.
2. Put in rice, garlic, turmeric, and cinnamon and cook, stirring often, until grain edges begin to turn translucent, approximately three minutes.
3. Mix in water and bring to simmer. Decrease heat to low, cover, and simmer gently until rice becomes soft and water is absorbed, 16 to 18 minutes.
4. Remove from the heat, drizzle currants over pilaf. Cover, laying clean dish towel underneath lid, and let pilaf sit for about ten minutes.
5. Put in almonds to pilaf and fluff gently with fork to combine. Sprinkle with salt and pepper to taste. Serve.

Nutrition:

- ✓ Calories: 180
- ✓ Carbs: 36g
- ✓ Fat: 2g
- ✓ Protein: 4g

Brown Rice Salad with Asparagus, Goat Cheese, and Lemon

Preparation time: 15 minutes

Cooking time: 35 minutes

Servings: 4-6

Ingredients:

- ¼ cup minced fresh parsley
- ¼ cup slivered almonds, toasted
- 1 pound asparagus, trimmed and cut into 1-inch lengths
- 1 shallot, minced
- 1 teaspoon grated lemon zest plus 3 tablespoons juice
- 1½ cups long-grain brown rice
- 2 ounces goat cheese, crumbled (½ cup)
- 3½ tablespoons extra-virgin olive oil
- Salt and pepper

Directions:

1. Bring 4 quarts water to boil in a Dutch oven. Put in rice and 1½ teaspoons salt and cook, stirring intermittently, until rice is tender, about half an hour.
2. Drain rice, spread onto rimmed baking sheet, and drizzle with 1 tablespoon lemon juice. Allow it to cool completely, about 15 minutes.
3. Heat 1 tablespoon oil in 12-inch frying pan on high heat until just smoking. Put in asparagus, ¼ teaspoon salt, and ¼ teaspoon pepper and cook, stirring intermittently, until asparagus is browned and crisp-tender, about 4 minutes; move to plate and allow to cool slightly.
4. Beat remaining 2½ tablespoons oil, lemon zest and remaining 2 tablespoons juice, shallot, ½ teaspoon salt, and ½ teaspoon pepper together in a big container.
5. Put in rice, asparagus, 2 tablespoons goat cheese, 3 tablespoons almonds, and 3 tablespoons parsley. Gently toss to combine and allow to sit for about 10 minutes.
6. Sprinkle with salt and pepper to taste. Move to serving platter and drizzle with remaining 2 tablespoons goat cheese, remaining 1 tablespoon almonds, and remaining 1 tablespoon parsley. Serve.

Nutrition:

- ✓ Calories: 197
- ✓ Carbs: 6g
- ✓ Fat: 16g
- ✓ Protein: 7g

Carrot-Almond-Bulgur Salad

Preparation time: 1 hour & 45 minutes

Cooking time: 0 minutes

Servings: 4-6

Ingredients:

- 1/8 teaspoon cayenne pepper
- 1/3 cup chopped fresh cilantro
- 1/3 cup chopped fresh mint
- 1/3 cup extra-virgin olive oil
- ½ cup sliced almonds, toasted
- ½ teaspoon ground cumin
- 1 cup water
- 1½ cups medium-grind bulgur, rinsed
- 3 scallions, sliced thin
- 4 carrots, peeled and shredded
- 6 tablespoons lemon juice (2 lemons)
- Salt and pepper

Directions:

1. Mix bulgur, water, ¼ cup lemon juice, and ¼ teaspoon salt in a container. Cover and allow to sit at room temperature until grains are softened and liquid is fully absorbed, about 1½ hours.
2. Beat remaining 2 tablespoons lemon juice, oil, cumin, cayenne, and ½ teaspoon salt together in a big container.
3. Put in bulgur, carrots, scallions, almonds, mint, and cilantro and gently toss to combine. Sprinkle with salt and pepper to taste. Serve.

Nutrition:

- ✓ Calories: 240
- ✓ Carbs: 54g
- ✓ Fat: 2g

Chickpea-Spinach-Bulgur

Preparation time: 15 minutes

Cooking time: 23 minutes

Servings: 4-6

Ingredients:

- ¾ cup chicken or vegetable broth
- ¾ cup water
- 1 (15-ounce) can chickpeas, rinsed
- 1 cup medium-grind bulgur, rinsed
- 1 onion, chopped fine
- 1 tablespoon lemon juice
- 2 tablespoons za'atar
- 3 garlic cloves, minced
- 3 ounces (3 cups) baby spinach, chopped
- 3 tablespoons extra-virgin olive oil
- Salt and pepper

Directions:

1. Heat 2 tablespoons oil in a big saucepan on moderate heat until it starts to shimmer. Put in onion and ½ teaspoon salt and cook till they become tender, approximately 5 minutes.
2. Mix in garlic and 1 tablespoon za'atar and cook until aromatic, approximately half a minute. Mix in bulgur, chickpeas, broth, and water and bring to simmer. Decrease heat to low, cover, and simmer gently until bulgur is tender, 16 to 18 minutes.
3. Remove from the heat, lay clean dish towel underneath lid and let bulgur sit for about ten minutes.
4. Put in spinach, lemon juice, remaining 1 tablespoon za'atar, and residual 1 tablespoon oil and fluff gently with fork to combine. Sprinkle with salt and pepper to taste. Serve.

Nutrition:

- ✓ Calories: 319
- ✓ Carbs: 43g
- ✓ Fat: 12g

Greek Farro Salad

Preparation time: 15 minutes

Cooking time: 20 minutes

Servings: 4

Ingredients:

Farro:

- ½ teaspoon fine-grain sea salt
- 1 cup farro, rinsed
- 1 tablespoon olive oil
- 2 garlic cloves, pressed or minced
- Salad:
- ½ small red onion, chopped and then rinsed under water to mellow the flavor
- 1 avocado, sliced into strips
- 1 cucumber, sliced into thin rounds
- 15 pitted Klamath olives, sliced into rounds
- 1-pint cherry tomatoes, sliced into rounds
- 2 cups cooked chickpeas (or one 14-ounce can, rinsed and drained)
- 5 ounces mixed greens
- Lemon wedges

Herbed Yogurt Ingredients:

- 1/8 teaspoon salt
- 1 ¼ cups plain Greek yogurt
- 1 ½ tablespoon lightly packed fresh dill, roughly chopped
- 1 ½ tablespoon lightly packed fresh mint, torn into pieces
- 1 tablespoon lemon juice (about ½ lemon)
- 1 tablespoon olive oil

Directions:

1. In a blender, blend and puree all herbed yogurt ingredients and set aside. Then cook the farro by placing in a pot filled halfway with water.
2. Bring to a boil, reduce fire to a simmer and cook for 15 minutes or until farro is tender. Drain well. Mix in salt, garlic, and olive oil and fluff to coat.
3. Evenly divide the cooled farro into 4 bowls. Evenly divide the salad ingredients on the 4 farro bowl. Top with ¼ of the yogurt dressing. Serve and enjoy.

Nutrition:

- ✓ Calories: 428
- ✓ Protein: 17.7g
- ✓ Carbs: 47.6g
- ✓ Fat: 24.5g

POULTRY AND MEAT RECIPES

Lemon-Garlic Chicken and Green Beans with Caramelized Onions

Preparation Time: 10 minutes

Cooking Time: 65 minutes

Servings: 2

Ingredients:

- 3 tbsp. Extra-virgin olive oil
- 3 tbsp. freshly squeezed lemon juice
- 2 tbsp. minced garlic
- 1 tsp. sea salt, plus additional for seasoning
- ¼ tsp. freshly ground black pepper
- ¼ tsp. paprika
- ⅛ tsp. red pepper flakes
- 2 large boneless, skinless free-range chicken breasts
- 1 yellow onion, quartered
- 2 cups trimmed green beans
- ¼ cup Golden Ghee, melted

Directions:

1. In .a medium bowl or a zipper-top plastic bag, combine the olive oil, lemon juice, garlic, salt, black pepper, paprika, and red pepper flakes.
2. Put the chicken then coat it in the marinade.
3. Cover the bowl or seal the bag then marinate the chicken in the fridge for at least 1 hour, or overnight if possible.
4. Preheat the oven to 350°F.
5. Dice 1 of the onion quarters, and cut the remaining 3 quarters into large chunks.
6. Put the larger chunks of onion across the bottom of a cast iron or ovenproof skillet.
7. Put the green beans, then scatter the diced onion above. Place on the top the green beans and onion with the ghee. Put the marinated chicken breasts on the green beans then spoon the remaining marinade at the chicken. Season the dish with a sprinkle of sea salt.
8. Bake the chicken until its internal temperature reaches at least 165°F, about 65 minutes. Serve hot.

Nutrition:

- ✓ Calories: 803
- ✓ Total Fat: 61g
- ✓ Saturated Fat: 23g
- ✓ Protein: 53g
- ✓ Cholesterol: 217mg
- ✓ Carbohydrates: 14g
- ✓ Fiber: 5g
- ✓ Net Carbs: 9g

Tarragon Chicken with Roasted Balsamic Turnips

Preparation Time: 10 minutes

Cooking Time: 50 minutes

Servings: 2-4

Ingredients:

- 1 pound chicken thighs
- 2 lb. turnips, cut into wedges
- 2 tbsp. olive oil
- 1 tbsp. balsamic vinegar
- 1 tbsp. tarragon
- Salt and black pepper, to taste

Directions:

1. Set the oven to 400°F then grease a baking dish with olive oil. Cook turnips in boiling water for 10 minutes, drain and set aside. Add the chicken and turnips to the baking dish.
2. Sprinkle with tarragon, black pepper, and salt. Roast for 35 minutes. Remove the baking dish, drizzle the turnip wedges with balsamic vinegar and return to the oven for another 5 minutes.

Nutrition:

- ✓ Calories: 383
- ✓ Fat: 26g
- ✓ Net Carbs: 9.5g
- ✓ Protein: 21.3g

Turmeric Chicken Wings with Ginger Sauce

Preparation Time: 5 minutes

Cooking Time: 20 minutes

Servings: 2-4

Ingredients:

- 2 tbsp. olive oil
- 1 pound chicken wings, cut in half
- 1 tbsp. turmeric
- 1 tbsp. cumin
- 3 tbsp. fresh ginger, grated
- Salt and black pepper, to taste
- Juice of ½ lime
- 1 cup thyme leaves
- ¾ cup cilantro, chopped
- 1 tbsp. water
- 1 jalapeño pepper

Directions:

1. In a bowl, stir together 1 tbsp. ginger, cumin, and salt, half of the olive oil, black pepper, turmeric, and cilantro. Place in the chicken wings pieces, toss to coat, and refrigerate for 20 minutes.
2. Heat the grill to high heat. Remove the wings from the marinade, drain, and grill for 20 minutes, turning from time to time, then set aside.
3. Using a blender, combine thyme, remaining ginger, salt, jalapeno pepper, black pepper, lime juice, the remaining olive oil, and water, and blend well. Serve the chicken wings topped with the sauce.

Nutrition:

- ✓ Calories 253
- ✓ Fat 16.1g
- ✓ Net Carbs 4.1g
- ✓ Protein 21.7g

Curry Chicken Lettuce Wraps

Preparation Time: 15 minutes

Cooking Time: 10 minutes

Servings: 5

Ingredients:

- 2 Minced garlic cloves
- 25 cups Minced onion
- 1 lb. Chicken thighs – skinless & boneless
- 2 tbsp. Ghee
- 1 tsp. Black pepper
- 2 tsp. Curry powder
- 1.5 tsp. Salt
- 1 cup Riced cauliflower
- 5-6 Lettuce leaves
- Keto-friendly sour cream (as desired - count the carbs)

Directions:

1. Mince the garlic and onions. Set aside for now.
2. Pull out the bones and skin from the chicken and dice into one-inch pieces.
3. On the stovetop, add 2 tbsp. of ghee to a skillet and melt. Toss in the onion and sauté until browned. Fold in the chicken and sprinkle with the garlic, pepper, and salt.
4. Cook for eight minutes. Stir in the remainder of the ghee, riced cauliflower, and curry. Stir until well mixed.
5. Prepare the lettuce leaves and add the mixture.
6. Serve with a dollop of cream.

Nutrition:

- ✓ Calories: 554
- ✓ Net Carbs: 7 g
- ✓ Total Fat Content: 36 g
- ✓ Protein: 50 g

Nacho Chicken Casserole

Preparation Time: 15 minutes

Cooking Time: 25 minutes

Servings: 6

Ingredients:

- 1 medium Jalapeño pepper
- 1.75lb. Chicken thighs
- Pepper and salt (to taste)
- 2 tbsp. Olive oil
- 1.5tsp. Chili seasoning
- 4 oz. Cheddar cheese
- 4 oz. Cream cheese
- 3 tbsp. Parmesan cheese
- 1 cup Green chilies and tomatoes
- .25 cup Sour cream
- 1 pkg. Frozen cauliflower
- Also Needed: Immersion blender

Directions:

1. Warm the oven to reach 375° Fahrenheit.
2. Slice the jalapeño into pieces and set aside.
3. Cutaway the skin and bones from the chicken. Chop it and sprinkle using the pepper and salt. Prepare in a skillet using a portion of olive oil on the med-high temperature setting until browned.
4. Mix in the sour cream, cream cheese, and ¾ of the cheddar cheese. Stir until melted and combined well. Place in the tomatoes and chilies. Stir then put it all to a baking dish.
5. Cook the cauliflower in the microwave. Blend in the rest of the cheese with the immersion blender until it resembles mashed potatoes. Season as desired.
6. Spread the cauliflower concoction over the casserole and sprinkle with the peppers. Bake approximately 15 to 20 minutes.

Nutrition:

- ✓ Calories: 426
- ✓ Net Carbs: 4.3 g
- ✓ Total Fat Content: 32.2 g
- ✓ Protein: 31 g

Pesto & Mozzarella Chicken Casserole

Preparation Time: 10 minutes

Cooking Time: 25-30 minutes

Servings: 8

Ingredients:

- Cooking oil (as needed)
- 2 lb. Grilled & cubed chicken breasts
- 8 oz. Cubed mozzarella
- 8 oz. Cream cheese
- 8 oz. Shredded mozzarella
- 25 cup Pesto

Directions:

1. Warm the oven to 400° Fahrenheit. Spritz a casserole dish with a spritz of cooking oil spray.
2. Combine the pesto, heavy cream, and softened cream cheese.
3. Add the chicken and cubed mozzarella into the greased dish.
4. Sprinkle the chicken using the shredded mozzarella. Bake for 25-30 minutes.

Nutrition:

- ✓ Calories: 451
- ✓ Net Carbs: 3 g
- ✓ Total Fat Content: 30 g
- ✓ Protein: 38 g

Chicken Quiche

Preparation Time: 15 minutes

Cooking Time: 50 minutes

Servings: 6

Ingredients:

- 16 oz. almond flour
- 7 medium eggs
- Salt and ground black pepper to taste
- 2 tbsp. coconut oil
- 1 lb. ground chicken
- 2 small zucchini, grated
- 1 tsp. dried oregano
- 1 tsp. fennel seeds
- ½ cup heavy cream

Directions:

1. Place almond flour, 1 egg, salt, and coconut oil in blender or food processor and blend.
2. Grease pie pan and pour the dough in it. Press well on the bottom.

3. Preheat pan on medium heat and toss ground chicken, cook for 2 minutes, set aside.
4. In a medium bowl, whisk together 6 eggs, zucchini, oregano, salt, pepper, fennel seeds, and heavy cream.
5. Add chicken to egg mixture and stir well.
6. Preheat oven to 350 F.
7. Pour egg mixture into pie pan and place in oven. Cook for 40 minutes.
8. Let it cool and slice. Serve.

Nutrition:

- ✓ Calories
- ✓ 295
- ✓ Carbs 3.95g
- ✓ Fat 24g
- ✓ Protein 19g

Chicken Parmigiana

Preparation Time: 15 minutes

Cooking Time: 26 minutes

Servings: 4

Ingredients:

- 1 large organic egg, beaten
- ½ cup of superfine blanched almond flour
- ¼ cup Parmesan cheese, grated
- ½ teaspoon dried parsley
- ½ teaspoon paprika
- ½ teaspoon garlic powder
- Salt and ground black pepper, as required
- 4 -6-ounces grass-fed skinless, boneless chicken breasts, pounded into a ½-inch thickness
- ¼ cup olive oil
- 1½ cups marinara sauce
- 4 ounces mozzarella cheese, thinly sliced
- 2 tablespoons fresh parsley, chopped

Directions:

1. Preheat the oven to 375 degrees F.
2. Add the beaten egg into a shallow dish.
3. Place the almond flour, Parmesan, parsley, spices, salt, and black pepper in another shallow dish and mix well.
4. Dip each chicken breast into the beaten egg and then coat with the flour mixture.

5. Heat the oil in a deep skillet over medium-high heat and fry the chicken breasts for about 3 minutes per side.
6. Using a slotted spoon, moved the chicken breasts onto a paper towel-lined plate to drain.
7. At the bottom of a casserole, put about ½ cup of marinara sauce and spread evenly.
8. Arrange the chicken breasts over marinara sauce in a single layer.
9. Top with the remaining marinara sauce, followed by mozzarella cheese slices.
10. Bake for about at least 20 minutes or until done completely.
11. Take off from the oven and serve hot with the garnishing of fresh parsley.

Nutrition:

- ✓ Calories: 542
- ✓ Net Carbs: 5.7g
- ✓ Carbohydrate: 9g
- ✓ Fiber: 3.3g
- ✓ Protein: 54.2g
- ✓ Fat: 33.2g
- ✓ Sugar: 3.8g
- ✓ Sodium: 609mg

Baked Chicken Meatballs - Habanero & Green Chili

Preparation Time: 10 minutes

Cooking Time: 25 minutes

Servings: 15

Ingredients:

- 1 pound ground chicken
- 1 poblano pepper
- 1 habanero pepper
- 1 jalapeno pepper
- 1/2 cup cilantro
- 1 tbsp. vinegar
- 1 tbsp. olive oil
- Salt to taste

Directions:

1. Preheat broiler to 400 degrees Fahrenheit.
2. In an enormous blending bowl, join chicken, minced peppers, cilantro, salt, and

vinegar with your hands. Structure 1-inch meatballs with the blend

3. Coat every meatball with olive oil, at that point, place on a rimmed heating sheet or meal dish.
4. Heat for 25 minutes

Nutrition:

- ✓ Calories 54
- ✓ Fat 3g
- ✓ Carbs 5g
- ✓ Protein 5g

Winter Chicken with Vegetables

Preparation Time: 5 minutes

Cooking Time: 30 minutes

Servings: 2

Ingredients:

- 2 tbsp. olive oil
- 2 cups whipping cream
- 1 pound chicken breasts, chopped
- 1 onion, chopped
- 1 carrot, chopped
- 2 cups chicken stock
- Salt and black pepper, to taste
- 1 bay leaf
- 1 turnip, chopped
- 1 parsnip, chopped
- 1 cup green beans, chopped
- 2 tsps. fresh thyme, chopped

Directions:

1. Heat a pan at medium heat and warm the olive oil. Sauté the onion for 3 minutes, pour in the stock, carrot, turnip, parsnip, chicken, and bay leaf. Place to a boil, and simmer for 20 minutes.
2. Add in the asparagus and cook for 7 minutes. Discard the bay leaf, stir in the whipping cream, adjust the seasoning, and scatter it with fresh thyme to serve.

Nutrition:

- ✓ Calories 483
- ✓ Fat 32.5g
- ✓ Net Carbs 6.9g

- ✓ Protein 33g

Paprika Chicken & Pancetta in a Skillet

Preparation Time: 20 minutes

Cooking Time: 10 minutes

Servings: 2

Ingredients:

- 1 tbsp. olive oil
- 5 pancetta strips, chopped
- 1/3 cup Dijon mustard
- Salt and black pepper, to taste
- 1 onion, chopped
- 1 cup chicken stock
- 2 chicken breasts, skinless and boneless
- ¼ tsp. sweet paprika
- 2 tbsp. oregano, chopped

Directions:

1. In a bowl, combine the paprika, black pepper, salt, and mustard. Sprinkle this mixture the chicken breasts and massage.
2. Heat a skillet over medium heat, stir in the pancetta, cook until it browns, for about 3-4 minutes, and remove to a plate.
3. To the pancetta fat, add olive oil and cook the chicken breasts for 2 minutes per side. Place in the stock, black pepper, pancetta, salt, and onion. Sprinkle with oregano and serve.

Nutrition:

- ✓ Calories 323
- ✓ Fat 21g
- ✓ Net Carbs 4.8g
- ✓ Protein 24.5g

Chili & Lemon Marinated Chicken Wings

Preparation Time: 5 minutes

Cooking Time: 12 minutes

Servings: 2-4

Ingredients:

- 3 tbsp. olive oil

- 1 tsp. coriander seeds
- 1 tsp. xylitol
- 1 pound wings
- Juice from 1 lemon
- ½ cup fresh parsley, chopped
- 2 garlic cloves, minced
- 1 red chili pepper, chopped
- Salt and black pepper, to taste
- Lemon wedges, for serving
- ½ tsp. cilantro

Directions:

1. Using a bowl, stir together lemon juice, xylitol, garlic, salt, red chili pepper, cilantro, olive oil, and black pepper. Place in the chicken wings and toss well to coat. Refrigerate for 2 hours.
2. Preheat grill over high heat. Add the chicken wings, and grill each side for 6 minutes. Serve the chicken wings with lemon wedges.
- ✓ Nutrition:
- ✓ Calories 223
- ✓ Fat 12g
- ✓ Net Carbs 5.1g
- ✓ Protein 16.8g

Cipollini & Bell Pepper Chicken Souvlaki

Preparation Time: 5 minutes

Cooking Time: 12 minutes

Servings: 2-4

Ingredients:

- 2 chicken breasts, cubed
- 2 tbsp. olive oil
- 2 cloves garlic, minced
- 1 red bell pepper, cut into chunks
- 8 oz. small cipollini
- ½ cup lemon juice
- Salt and black pepper to taste
- 1 tsp. rosemary leaves to garnish
- 2 to 4 lemon wedges to garnish

Directions:

1. Thread the chicken, bell pepper, and cipollini onto skewers and set aside. In a

bowl, mix half of the oil, garlic, salt, black pepper, and lemon juice, and add the chicken skewers. Cover the bowl and let the chicken marinate for at least 2 hours in the refrigerator.
2. Preheat a grill to high heat and grill the skewers for 6 minutes on each side. Remove and serve garnished with rosemary leaves and lemons wedges.

Nutrition:

- ✓ Calories 363
- ✓ Fat 14.2g
- ✓ Net Carbs 4.2g
- ✓ Protein 32.5g

Pulled Buffalo Chicken Salad with Blue Cheese

Preparation Time: 10 minutes

Cooking Time: 30 minutes

Servings: 2

Ingredients:

- 2 boneless, skinless free-range chicken breasts
- 4 uncured center-cut bacon strips
- ¼ cup Buffalo Sauce
- 4 cups chopped romaine lettuce, divided
- ½ cup blue cheese dressing, divided
- ½ cup crumbled organic blue cheese, divided
- ¼ cup chopped red onion, divided

Directions:

1. Place a large pot of water to a boil over high heat.
2. Put the chicken breasts to the water, lower the heat then simmer the breasts until their internal temperature reaches 180°F, about 30 minutes.
3. Take the chicken to a bowl and let it cool for about 10 minutes.
4. On the other hand, crisp the bacon strips in a skillet over medium heat, about 3 minutes per side. Drain the bacon on a paper towel.
5. Shred the chicken using a fork and toss it with the buffalo sauce.

6. Divide the lettuce into 2 bowls. Top each with half of the pulled chicken, half of the blue cheese dressing, blue cheese crumbles, and chopped red onion. Crumble the bacon over the salads and serve.

Nutrition:

- ✓ Calories: 843
- ✓ Total Fat: 65g
- ✓ Saturated Fat: 14g
- ✓ Protein: 59g
- ✓ Cholesterol: 156mg
- ✓ Carbohydrates: 6g
- ✓ Fiber: 1g
- ✓ Net Carbs: 5g

Red Pepper and Mozzarella-Stuffed Chicken Caprese

Preparation Time: 10 minutes

Cooking Time: 40 minutes

Servings: 2

Ingredients:

- 2 tablespoons extra-virgin olive oil
- 2 chicken breasts, butterflied
- 10 fresh basil leaves
- 1 (8-ounce) ball mozzarella cheese, cut into 4 pieces
- 1 cup Roasted Red Peppers
- 2 tablespoons Italian seasoning
- Sea salt
- Freshly ground black pepper

Directions:

1. Preheat the oven to 400°F.
2. Line a rimmed baking sheet using a parchment paper.
3. Place 5 basil leaves inside each chicken breast.
4. Place 2 mozzarella slices inside each breast.
5. Divide the roasted red peppers into 2 breasts. Sprinkle the Italian seasoning generously over each breast and season them with salt and pepper. Close each breast to envelop the filling.

6. Put the breasts on the baking sheet and bake until cooked through about 40 minutes. Serve hot.

Nutrition:

- ✓ Calories: 539
- ✓ Total Fat: 30g
- ✓ Saturated Fat: 5g
- ✓ Protein: 63g
- ✓ Cholesterol 152mg
- ✓ Carbohydrates: 4g
- ✓ Fiber: 1g
- ✓ Net Carbs: 3g

Turnip Greens & Artichoke Chicken

Preparation Time: 5 minutes

Cooking Time: 30 minutes

Servings: 2

Ingredients:

- 4 ounces cream cheese
- 2 chicken breasts
- 4 oz. canned artichoke hearts, chopped
- 1 cup turnip greens
- ¼ cup Pecorino cheese, grated
- ½ tbsp. onion powder
- ½ tbsp. garlic powder
- Salt and black pepper, to taste
- 2 ounces Monterrey Jack cheese, shredded

Directions:

1. Line a baking dish using parchment paper and place it in the chicken breasts. Season with black pepper and salt. Set in the oven at 350 F and bake for 35 minutes.
2. In a bowl, combine the artichokes with onion powder, Pecorino cheese, salt, turnip greens, cream cheese, garlic powder, and black pepper. Take off the chicken from the oven, cut each piece in half, divide artichokes mixture on top, spread with Monterrey cheese, and bake for 5 more minutes.

Nutrition:

- ✓ Calories 443
- ✓ Fat 24.5g
- ✓ Net Carbs 4.2g

✓ Protein 35.4g

VEGETABLES AND VEGAN RECIPES

Lentils with Tomatoes and Turmeric

Preparation Time: 10 minutes

Cooking Time: 10 minutes

Servings: 4

Ingredients:

- 2 tbsp. Extra Olive Virgin Oil, plus extra for garnish
- 1 Onion, finely chopped
- 1 tbsp. Ground turmeric
- 1 tsp. Garlic powder
- 1 (14 oz.) can Lentils, drained
- 1 (14 oz.) can Chopped tomatoes, drained
- ½ tsp. Sea salt
- ¼ tsp. Freshly ground black pepper

Directions:

1. In a huge pot on medium-high heat, warm the olive oil until it shimmers.
2. Add the onion and turmeric, and cook for about 5 minutes, occasionally stirring, until soft.
3. Add the garlic powder, lentils, tomatoes, salt, and pepper. Cook for 5 minutes, stirring occasionally. Serve garnished with additional olive oil, if desired

Nutrition:

- ✓ Calories: 24
- ✓ Total Fat: 8g
- ✓ Total Carbs: 34g
- ✓ Sugar: 5g
- ✓ Fiber: 15g
- ✓ Protein: 12g
- ✓ Sodium 243mg

Whole-Wheat Pasta with Tomato-Basil Sauce

Preparation Time: 15 minutes

Cooking Time: 10 minutes

Servings: 4

Ingredients:

- 2 tbsp. Extra Olive virgin oil
- 1 Onion, minced
- 6 Garlic cloves, minced
- 2 (28 oz.) can crushed tomatoes, untrained
- ½ tsp. Sea salt
- ¼ tsp. Ground black pepper
- ¼ cup Basil leaves, chopped
- 1 (8 oz.) Package whole-wheat pasta

Directions:

1. In a huge pot on medium-high heat, warm the olive oil until it shimmers.
2. Add the onion. Cook for about 5 minutes, occasionally stirring, until soft.
3. Add the garlic. Cook for 30 seconds, stirring constantly.
4. Stir in the tomatoes, salt, and pepper. Bring it to a simmer. Reduce the heat to medium and cook for 5 minutes, stirring occasionally.
5. Pull it out from the heat then stir in the basil. Toss with the pasta.

Nutrition:

- ✓ Calories: 330
- ✓ Total Fat: 8g
- ✓ Total Carbs: 56g
- ✓ Sugar: 24g
- ✓ Fiber: 17g
- ✓ Protein: 14g
- ✓ Sodium: 1,000mg

Nutty and Fruity Garden Salad

Preparation Time: 10 minutes

Cooking Time: 0 minutes

Servings: 2

Ingredients:

- 6 cups baby spinach
- ½ cup chopped walnuts, toasted
- 1 ripe red pear, sliced
- 1 ripe persimmon, sliced
- 1 teaspoon garlic minced
- 1 shallot, minced
- 1 tablespoon extra-virgin olive oil
- 2 tablespoons fresh lemon juice
- 1 teaspoon wholegrain mustard

Directions:

1. Mix well garlic, shallot, oil, lemon juice, and mustard in a large salad bowl.
2. Add spinach, pear, and persimmon. Toss to coat well.
3. To serve, garnish with chopped pecans.

Nutrition:

- ✓ Calories 332
- ✓ Total Fat 21g
- ✓ Saturated Fat 2g
- ✓ Total Carbs 37g
- ✓ Net Carbs 28g
- ✓ Protein 7g
- ✓ Sugar: 20g
- ✓ Fiber 9g
- ✓ Sodium 75mg
- ✓ Potassium 864mg

Roasted Root Vegetables

Preparation Time: 10 minutes

Cooking Time: 1 hour and 30 minutes

Servings: 6

Ingredients:

- 2 tbsp. olive oil
- 1 head garlic, cloves separated and peeled
- 1 large turnip, peeled and cut into ½-inch pieces
- 1 medium-sized red onion, cut into ½-inch pieces
- 1 ½ lb. beets, trimmed but not peeled, scrubbed and cut into ½-inch pieces
- 1 ½ lb. Yukon gold potatoes, unpeeled, cut into ½-inch pieces
- 2 ½ lbs. butternut squash, peeled, seeded, cut into ½-inch pieces

Directions:

1. Grease 2 rimmed and large baking sheets. Preheat oven to 425oF.
2. In a huge bowl, mix all ingredients thoroughly.
3. Into the two baking sheets, evenly divide the root vegetables, spread in one layer.
4. Season generously with pepper and salt.
5. Place it into the oven, then roast for at least 1 hour and 15 minutes or until golden brown and tender.
6. Remove from the oven and let it cool for at least 15 minutes before serving.

Nutrition:

- ✓ Calories 278
- ✓ Total Fat 5g,
- ✓ Saturated Fat 1g
- ✓ Total Carbs 57g
- ✓ Net Carbs 47g
- ✓ Protein 6g
- ✓ Sugar: 15g
- ✓ Fiber 10g
- ✓ Sodium 124mg
- ✓ Potassium 1598mg

Braised Kale

Preparation Time: 10 minutes

Cooking Time: 15 minutes

Servings: 3

Ingredients:

- 2 to 3 tbsp. water
- 1 tbsp. coconut oil
- ½ sliced red pepper
- 2 stalk celery (sliced to ¼-inch thick)
- 5 cups of chopped kale

Directions:

1. Heat a pan over medium heat.
2. Add coconut oil and sauté the celery for at least five minutes.
3. Add the kale and red pepper.
4. Add a tablespoon of water.
5. Let the vegetables wilt for a few minutes. Add a tablespoon of water if the kale starts to stick to the pan.
6. Serve warm.

Nutrition:

- ✓ Calories 61
- ✓ Total Fat 5g
- ✓ Saturated Fat 1g
- ✓ Total Carbs 3g
- ✓ Net Carbs 2g
- ✓ Protein 1g
- ✓ Sugar: 1g
- ✓ Fiber 1g
- ✓ Sodium 20mg
- ✓ Potassium 185mg

Braised Leeks, Cauliflower and Artichoke Hearts

Preparation Time: 10 minutes

Cooking Time: 10 minutes

Servings: 4

Ingredients:

- 2 tbsp. coconut oil
- 2 garlic cloves, chopped
- 1 ½ cup artichoke hearts
- 1 ½ cups chopped leeks
- 1 ½ cups cauliflower flowerets

Directions:

1. In a skillet, warm oil on medium-high heat temperature.
2. Put the garlic and sauté for one minute. Add the vegetables and constantly stir until the vegetables are cooked.
3. Serve with roasted chicken, fish or pork.

Nutrition:

- ✓ Calories 111
- ✓ Total Fat 7g
- ✓ Saturated Fat 1g
- ✓ Total Carbs 12g

- ✓ Net Carbs 8g
- ✓ Protein 3g
- ✓ Sugar: 2g
- ✓ Fiber 4g
- ✓ Sodium 65mg
- ✓ Potassium 305mg

Celery Root Hash Browns

Preparation Time: 10 minutes

Cooking Time: 10 minutes

Servings: 4

Ingredients:

- 4 tbsp. coconut oil
- ½ tsp. sea salt
- 2 to 3 medium celery roots

Directions:

1. Scrub the celery root clean and peel it using a vegetable peeler.
2. Grate the celery root in a manual grater.
3. In a skillet, add oil and heat it over medium heat.
4. Place the grated celery root on the skillet and sprinkle with salt.
5. Let it cook for 10 minutes on each side or until the grated celery turns brown.
6. Serve warm.

Nutrition:

- ✓ Calories 160
- ✓ Total Fat 14g
- ✓ Saturated Fat 3g
- ✓ Total Carbs 10g
- ✓ Net Carbs 7g
- ✓ Protein 1.5g
- ✓ Sugar: 0g
- ✓ Fiber 3g
- ✓ Sodium 314mg
- ✓ Potassium 320mg

Braised Carrots 'n Kale

Preparation Time: 10 minutes

Cooking Time: 10 minutes

Servings: 2

Ingredients:

- 1 tablespoon coconut oil
- 1 onion, sliced thinly
- 5 cloves of garlic, minced
- 3 medium carrots, sliced thinly
- 10 ounces of kale, chopped
- ½ cup water
- Salt and pepper to taste
- A dash of red pepper flakes

Directions:

1. Warm oil in a skillet over medium flame and sauté the onion and garlic until fragrant.
2. Toss in the carrots and stir for 1 minute. Add the kale and water. Season with salt and pepper to taste.
3. Close the lid and allow to simmer for 5 minutes.
4. Sprinkle with red pepper flakes.
5. Serve and enjoy.

Nutrition:

- ✓ Calories 161
- ✓ Total Fat 8g
- ✓ Saturated Fat 1g
- ✓ Total Carbs 20g
- ✓ Net Carbs 14g
- ✓ Protein 8g
- ✓ Sugar: 6g
- ✓ Fiber 6g
- ✓ Sodium 63mg
- ✓ Potassium 900mg

Cauliflower Fritters

Preparation Time: 10 minutes

Cooking Time: 15 minutes

Servings: 6

Ingredients:

- 1 large cauliflower head, cut into florets
- 2 eggs, beaten
- ½ teaspoon turmeric
- ½ teaspoon salt
- ¼ teaspoon black pepper
- 1 tablespoon coconut oil

Directions:

1. Put the cauliflower florets in a pot with water and bring to a boil. Cook until tender, around 5 minutes of boiling. Drain well.
2. Place the cauliflower, eggs, turmeric, salt, and pepper into the food processor.
3. Pulse until the mixture becomes coarse.
4. Transfer into a bowl. Using your hands, form six small flattened balls and place in the fridge for at least 1 hour until the mixture hardens.
5. Warm the oil in a nonstick pan and fry the cauliflower patties for 3 minutes on each side.
6. Serve and enjoy.

Nutrition:

- ✓ Calories 53
- ✓ Total Fat 6g
- ✓ Saturated Fat 2g
- ✓ Total Carbs 2
- ✓ Net Carbs 1g
- ✓ Protein 3g
- ✓ Sugar: 1g
- ✓ Fiber 1g
- ✓ Sodium 228mg
- ✓ Potassium 159mg

Sweet Potato Puree

Preparation Time: 10 minutes

Cooking Time: 15 minutes

Servings: 5

Ingredients:

- 2 pounds sweet potatoes, peeled
- 1 ½ cups water
- 5 Medjool dates, pitted and chopped

Directions:

1. Place water and potatoes in a pot.
2. Close the lid and boil for at least 15 minutes until the potatoes are soft.
3. Drain the potatoes and place them in a food processor together with the dates.
4. Pulse until smooth.
5. Serve and enjoy.

Nutrition:

- ✓ Calories 172
- ✓ Total Fat 0.2g
- ✓ Saturated Fat 0g
- ✓ Total Carbs 41g
- ✓ Net Carbs 36g
- ✓ Protein 3g
- ✓ Sugar: 14g
- ✓ Fiber 5g
- ✓ Sodium 10mg
- ✓ Potassium 776mg

Vegetable Potpie

Preparation Time: 10 minutes

Cooking Time: 10 minutes

Servings: 8

Ingredients:

- 1 recipe pastry for double-crust pie
- 2 tbsps. cornstarch
- 1 tsp. ground black pepper
- 1 tsp. kosher salt
- 3 cups vegetable broth
- 1 cup fresh green beans, snapped into ½ inch
- 2 cups cauliflower florets
- 2 stalks celery, sliced ¼ inch wide
- 2 potatoes, peeled and diced
- 2 large carrots, diced
- 1 clove garlic, minced
- 8 oz. mushroom
- 1 onion, chopped
- 2 tbsp. olive oil

Directions:

1. In a large saucepan, sauté garlic in oil until lightly browned, add onions and continue sautéing until soft and translucent.
2. Add celery, potatoes, and carrots and sauté for 3 minutes.
3. Add vegetable broth, green beans, and cauliflower and bring to a boil. Slow fire and simmer until vegetables are slightly tender. Season with pepper and salt.
4. Mix ¼ cup water and cornstarch in a small bowl. Stir until the mixture is smooth and has no lumps. Then pour into the vegetable pot while mixing constantly.

5. Continue mixing until soup thickens, around 3 minutes. Remove from fire.
6. Meanwhile, roll out pastry dough and place on an oven-safe 11x7 baking dish. Pour the vegetable filling and then cover with another pastry dough. Seal and flute the edges of the dough and prick the top dough with a fork in several places.
7. Bake the dish in a preheated oven of 425oF for 30 minutes or until the crust has turned a golden brown.

Nutrition:

- ✓ Calories 202
- ✓ Total Fat 10g
- ✓ Saturated Fat 2g
- ✓ Total Carbs 26g
- ✓ Net Carbs 23g
- ✓ Protein 4g
- ✓ Sugar: 3g
- ✓ Fiber 3g
- ✓ Sodium 466m
- ✓ Potassium 483mg

Fruit Bowl with Yogurt Topping

Preparation Time: 15 minutes

Cooking Time: 0 minutes

Servings: 6

Ingredients:

- ¼ cup golden brown sugar
- 2/3 cup minced fresh ginger
- 1 16-oz Greek yogurt
- ¼ tsp. ground cinnamon
- 2 tbsp. honey
- ½ cup dried cranberries
- 3 navel oranges
- 2 large tangerines
- 1 pink grapefruit, peeled

Directions:

1. Into sections, break tangerines and grapefruit.
2. Slice tangerine sections in half and grapefruit sections into thirds. Place all sliced fruits and its juices in a large bowl.
3. Peel oranges, remove the pith, slice into ¼-inch thick rounds, and then cut into

quarters. Transfer to the bowl of fruit along with juices. In a bowl, add cinnamon, honey, and ¼ cup of cranberries. Place in the ref for an hour. In a medium bowl, mix ginger and yogurt. Place on top of the fruit bowl, drizzle with remaining cranberries and brown sugar.

4. Serve and enjoy.

Nutrition:

- ✓ Calories 171 Fat 1g
- ✓ Carbs 35g
- ✓ Protein 9g
- ✓ Fiber 3g

Collard Green Wrap

Preparation Time: 10 minutes

Cooking Time: 0 minutes

Servings: 4

Ingredients:

- ½ block feta, cut into 4 (1-inch thick) strips (4-oz)
- ½ cup purple onion, diced
- ½ medium red bell pepper, julienned
- 1 medium cucumber, julienned
- 4 large cherry tomatoes, halved
- 4 large collard green leaves, washed
- 8 whole kalamata olives, halved

Sauce Ingredients:

- 1 cup low-fat plain Greek yogurt
- 1 tablespoon white vinegar
- 1 teaspoon garlic powder
- 2 tablespoons minced fresh dill
- 2 tablespoons olive oil
- 2.5-ounces cucumber, seeded and grated (¼-whole)
- Salt and pepper to taste

Directions:

1. Make the sauce first: make sure to squeeze out all the excess liquid from the cucumber after grating. In a small bowl, put all together the sauce ingredients and mix thoroughly then refrigerate.
2. Prepare and slice all wrap ingredients.

3. On a flat surface, spread one collard green leaf. Spread 2 tablespoons of Tzatziki sauce in the middle of the leaf.
4. Layer ¼ of each of the tomatoes, feta, olives, onion, pepper, and cucumber. Place them on the center of the leaf, like piling them high instead of spreading them.
5. Fold the leaf-like you would a burrito. Repeat process for remaining ingredients.
6. Serve and enjoy.

Nutrition:

- ✓ Calories 463
- ✓ Fat 31g
- ✓ Carbs 31g
- ✓ Protein 20g
- ✓ Fiber 7g

Wild Rice with Spicy Chickpeas

Preparation Time: 15 minutes

Cooking Time: 60 minutes

Servings: 6-7

Ingredients:

- 1 Cup basmati rice
- 1 Cup wild rice
- Salt & pepper to taste
- 4 tbsps. Olive oil
- 1 tbsp. Garlic powder
- 2 tsps. cumin powder
- ¼ Cup sunflower oil
- 3 Cups chickpeas
- 1 tsp. Flour
- 1 tsp. Curry powder
- 3 tsps. Paprika powder
- 1 tsp. Dill
- 3 tbsps. parsley (chopped)
- 1 Medium onion (thinly sliced)
- 2 Cups currants

Directions:

1. For cooking wild rice, fill the half pot with water and bring it to boil. Put the rice and let it simmer for at least 40 minutes.
2. Take olive in the pot and heat it on medium flame. Now add cumin powder,

salt, and water and bring it to boil. Then add basmati rice and cook for 20 minutes.

3. Leave rice for cooking and prepare spicy chickpeas. Heat 2tbsp of olive oil in the pan and toss chickpeas, garlic powder, salt & pepper, cumin, and paprika powder in it.
4. In another pan, cook onion with sunflower oil until it is golden brown and add flour.
5. Mix flour and onion with your hands.
6. For serving, place both types of rice in a bowl with spicy chickpeas and fry the onion. Garnish it with parsley and herbs.

Nutrition:

- ✓ Calories: 647 kcal
- ✓ Protein: 25.43 g
- ✓ Fat: 25.72 g
- ✓ Carbohydrates: 88.3 g

Mashed Cauliflower

Preparation Time: 10 minutes

Cooking Time: 10 minutes

Servings: 3

Ingredients:

- 1 cauliflower head
- 1 tablespoon olive oil
- ½ tsp. salt
- ¼ tsp. dill
- Pepper to taste
- 2 tbsps. low-fat milk

Directions:

1. Place a small pot of water to a boil.
2. Chop cauliflower in florets.
3. Add florets to boiling water and boil uncovered for 5 minutes. Turn off fire and let it sit for 5 minutes more.
4. In a blender, add all ingredients except for cauliflower and blend to mix well.
5. Drain cauliflower well and add it to a blender. Puree until smooth and creamy.
6. Serve and enjoy.

Nutrition:

- ✓ Calories 78
- ✓ Fat 5g
- ✓ Carbs 6g

- ✓ Protein 2g
- ✓ Fiber 2g

Cashew Pesto & Parsley with veggies

Preparation Time: 15 minutes

Cooking Time: 10 minutes

Servings: 3-4

Ingredients:

- 3 Zucchini (sliced)
- 8 Soaked bamboo skewers
- 2 Red capsicums
- ¼Cup olive oil
- 750grams Eggplant
- 4 Lemon cheeks

For Serving

- Couscous salad

For Preparing Cashew Pesto

- ½Cup cashew (roasted)
- ½ Cup parsley
- 2 Cups of grated parmesan
- 2 tbsps. Lime juice
- ¼Cup olive oil

Directions:

1. Toss capsicum, eggplant, and zucchini with oil and salt and thread it onto skewers.
2. Cook bamboo sticks for 6-8 minutes on a barbecue grill pan on medium heat.
3. Also, grill lemon cheeks from both sides.
4. For preparing cashew pesto, combine all ingredients in the food processor and blend.
5. For serving, place grill skewers in a plate with grill lemon slices and drizzle some cashew pesto over it.

Nutrition:

- ✓ Calories: 666 kcal
- ✓ Protein: 23.96 g
- ✓ Fat: 48.04 g
- ✓ Carbohydrates: 41.4 g

Spicy Chickpeas with Roasted Vegetables

Preparation Time: 10 minutes

Cooking Time: 25 minutes

Servings: 2-3

Ingredients:

- 1 Large carrot (peeled)
- 2 tbsps. Sunflower oil
- 1 Cauliflower head
- 1tbsp ground cumin
- ½ Red onions (diced)
- 1 Red pepper (deseeded)
- 400g Can chickpeas

Directions:

1. Line a large baking tine in the preheated oven (at 240C).
2. Cut all the vegetables and toss with salt, pepper, and onion.
3. In a bowl, whisk olive oil, pepper, and cumin powder.
4. Add all veggies in the bowl and toss.
5. Transfer vegetables on baking tin and baked it almost for 15 minutes.
6. Now add chickpeas and stir.
7. Return to the oven and bake it for the next 10 minutes.
8. Serve it with toast bread.

Nutrition:

- ✓ Calories: 348 kcal
- ✓ Protein: 14.29 g
- ✓ Fat: 15.88 g
- ✓ Carbohydrates: 40.65 g

Special Vegetable Kitchree

Preparation Time: 10 minutes

Cooking Time: 46 minutes

Servings: 5-6

Ingredients:

- ½Cup brown grain rice
- 1 Cup dry lentil or split peas
- 1tsp Sea salt, cumin powder, ground turmeric, ground fenugreek, and ground coriander
- 3 tbsps. Coconut oil
- 1 tbsp. Ginger
- 5 Cups vegetable stock
- 1 Cup baby spinach
- 1 Medium Zucchini (roughly chopped)
- 1 Small crown broccoli (chopped)
- Greek Yogurt (for serving)

Directions:

1. In a saucepan, warm the coconut oil on medium flame and add ginger, cumin, coriander, fennel seeds, fenugreek, and turmeric and cook it for 1 minute.
2. Now add lentils and brown rice in the spices and stir. Pour the vegetable stock in it and simmer for 40 minutes.
3. Add broccoli in the tender rice and lentils and cook for another 5 minutes. Now add other vegetables and stir for 10 minutes.
4. For serving, pour some Greek yogurt over vegetable kitcheree and serve hot.

Nutrition:

- ✓ Calories: 1728 kcal
- ✓ Protein: 4.13 g
- ✓ Fat: 190.35 g
- ✓ Carbohydrates: 17.31 g

Mashed Sweet Potato Burritos

Preparation Time: 15 minutes

Cooking Time: 60 minutes

Servings: 4

Ingredients:

- 4 Tortillas
- 1 Avocado
- 1 tsp. Capsicum, paprika powder, and oregano
- Salt & pepper as needed
- ½Cup sour cream
- 1 Can diced tomato
- 2 Sweet Potatoes (mashed)
- 2 Garlic cloves (minced)

- 1 tbsp. Cumin powder
- Fresh cilantro or parsley

Directions:

1. Before mashing roast sweet potatoes for 45 minutes in an already preheated (at 160°C) oven.
2. Cook onion in a frying pan with oil on medium heat. Add garlic cloves and cook for 1 minute.
3. Add 1 tin of tomatoes and leave it to simmer for 10 minutes. In halfway through, add salt & pepper, paprika, cumin powder, and black beans.
4. After 5 minutes, add avocado in it.
5. Now make burritos, mix one scoop of mashed potatoes with avocado filling.
6. Wrap your tortilla and grill it in the oven at 200C for 30seconds.
7. Serve it with sour cream and hot sauce.

Nutrition:

- ✓ Calories: 442 kcal
- ✓ Protein: 12.05 g
- ✓ Fat: 15.43 g
- ✓ Carbohydrates: 66.85 g

Toasted Cumin Crunch

Preparation Time: 10 minutes

Cooking Time: 1 minute

Servings: 1

Ingredients:

- 1 tbsp. Ground cumin seeds (Use pestle and mortar or Blender)
- 2 tbsp. Extra virgin olive oil
- 1 tsp. Crack black peppercorns
- ½ tsp. Cumin seeds, whole
- 1 tsp. Cilantro, finely chopped
- 1/2 Jalapeno, finely chopped
- 2 cups Green Cabbage, sliced
- 2 cups Carrots, grated
- ½ cup of Cilantro, chopped
- 3 tbsps. Lime Juice

Directions:

1. Get a large saucepan, and then heat the oil over medium heat.

2. Cook the peppercorns, coriander, and the whole cumin seeds for about a minute until browned.
3. Add in the jalapeno and then cook for another 45 seconds until tender.
4. Add in then the carrots and the cabbage, cooking for about 5 minutes or until the cabbage starts to soften.
5. Add in the crushed cumin seeds and cook for 30 seconds before taking off the heat and then stirring in the lime juice and the cilantro.
6. Serve warm.

Nutrition:

- ✓ Calories: 377 kcal
- ✓ Protein: 12.77 g
- ✓ Fat: 20.54 g
- ✓ Carbohydrates: 41.82 g

Light Mushroom Risotto

Preparation Time: 10 minutes

Cooking Time: 35 minutes

Servings: 4

Ingredients:

- 500g medium potatoes
- 300 g of mushrooms
- 250 g of arborous rice or carnaroli
- 1 onion
- 1 clove garlic
- 1 l of vegetable broth
- 1glass of white wine
- 50 g of Parmesan cheese
- 4 tablespoons of olive oil
- A sprig of parsley
- Salt and pepper

Directions:

1. Heat the vegetable broth. Put the vegetable broth to heat. Wash the parsley, potatoes, dry it, reserve some whole leaves for decorating, and chopping the rest. Grate the Parmesan cheese.
2. Poach the garlic and onion. Peel and clean the garlic and onion and chop them. In a

42

casserole with olive oil, beat them for about 5 minutes or so over low heat.

3. Skip the mushrooms. Meanwhile, clean the mushrooms. Leave a few whole pieces for decoration and the rest of the pieces in small pieces. Add them all to the casserole and sauté everything around five more minutes.

4. Incorporate the rice. Once you have sautéed the mushrooms with the onion and garlic, remove the ones that you had left whole and reserve them. Add the rice to the pan, arborous rice or carnaroli, and then sauté everything together for another 5 minutes, stirring constantly.

5. Make the risotto. Pour the glass of white wine and a broth of broth, and cook for 15 minutes, stirring frequently, and adding broth as the rice absorbs it.

6. Complete the risotto. After the indicated time, add the cheese, parsley, salt and pepper to taste, and the rest of the broth and cook for three more minutes, stirring vigorously. Let stand for 2 minutes and serve.

Nutrition:

- ✓ Calories: 111
- ✓ Total Fat: 2g
- ✓ Carbohydrates: 19g
- ✓ Fiber: 0 g
- ✓ Sugar: 18 g

Vegetable Pie

Preparation Time: 10 minutes

Cooking Time: 40 minutes

Servings: 6-8

Ingredients:

- 1 red pepper (you can make it green)
- 1 bunch parsley
- 1/2 grated carrot
- 6 mushrooms cut it into slices
- 6 eggs
- 1 tablespoon oil
- 1 teaspoon salt, one pepper and a small cup of bread crumbs

Directions:

1. First of all, put to heat the oven to 18oF.
2. You must cut everything in small squares (parsley) the carrot, the mushrooms cut in sheets ah, and use natural, but everything is to your liking you can use the pot.
3. Once you have everything cut, put a small piece of oil and put it in a pan to brown (all the vegetables).
4. Once the vegetables are golden brown, put the six eggs in a bowl, salt, pepper, and bread crumbs.
5. Put the vegetables in the mold (or muffin molds) to taste and the time of each one, pour the ingredients of the bowl and put it in the oven for 35 or 40 minutes.
6. Serve and enjoy.

Nutrition:

- ✓ Calories: 127 kcal
- ✓ Protein: 7.81 g
- ✓ Fat: 9.74 g
- ✓ Carbohydrates: 1.77 g

Turmeric Nachos

Preparation Time: 5 minutes

Cooking Time: 20-30 minutes

Servings: 2-3

Ingredients:

- 1 cup Cornmeal
- ½ cup Flour
- 1/4 teaspoon turmeric powder
- 1/4 teaspoon Aji wine
- Water as needed
- 2 tablespoons Oil

Directions:

1. Put cornmeal and flour in a bowl.
2. Add salt, turmeric powder, and aji wine.
3. Mix everything very well.
4. Now knead the dough firmly with warm water.
5. Cover the dough and leave it for 10-15 minutes to harden.
6. Grease your hands with a small amount of oil and knead the dough again.
7. Make a ball with the dough.
8. Take the ball and round it.

9. Push it a little and place it on the rolling board.
10. It grows a little like Chapatti.
11. After placing the poor, stab it with the help of a fork.
12. Then cut in half from the center and repeat the process.
13. Heat the oil in a deep pan and fry nachos over medium heat.
14. After this, lift the tip continuously. Stir until golden.
15. On the other hand, chips from other dough balls are also prepared.
16. When finished, drain the chip on the paper to remove excess oil. Allow the tip to cool completely.
17. Then put the fries on a plate and put the grated cheese, finely chopped onion, finely chopped tomatoes, and mayonnaise on top of the fries.

Nutrition:

- ✓ Calories: 378 kcal
- ✓ Protein: 8.03 g
- ✓ Fat: 12.22 g
- ✓ Carbohydrates: 57.66 g

Rucola Salad

Preparation Time: 10 minutes

Cooking Time: 0 minutes

Servings: 2

Ingredients:

- 4 teaspoons fresh lemon juice
- 4 teaspoons walnut oil
- low sodium salt and freshly ground pepper
- 6 cups rucola leaves and tender stems (about 6 ounces)
- Garlic powder to taste

Directions:

1. Put the lemon juice into a bowl. Gradually whisk in the oil. Season with low sodium salt and pepper.
2. Add the greens, toss until evenly dressed, and serve at once. This is delicious, and

feel free to add tomatoes or grated carrot and onion slices.
3. Substitution: Any mild green, such as lamb's lettuce, will do.

Nutrition:

- ✓ Calories: 163 kcal
- ✓ Protein: 9.16 g
- ✓ Fat: 12.94 g
- ✓ Carbohydrates: 5.92 g

Tasty Spring Salad

Preparation Time: 10 minutes

Cooking Time: 0 minutes

Servings: 2

Ingredients:

- 5 cups of any salad greens in the season of your choice
- Dressing:
- 125 mL (1/2 cup) olive oil
- 45 mL (3 tbsp.) lemon juice
- 15 mL (1 tbsp.) pure mustard powder
- 45 mL (3 tbsp.) capers, minced (optional)
- low sodium salt
- Pepper

Directions:

1. Combine salad greens and any other raw vegetables of choice.
2. Combine oil, lemon juice, and mustard. Mix well.
3. Add capers, low sodium salt, and pepper to taste.
4. Pour dressing over salad, toss and serve.

Nutrition:

- ✓ Calories: 2140 kcal
- ✓ Protein: 4.8 g
- ✓ Fat: 234.59 g
- ✓ Carbohydrates: 3.96 g

Pure Delish Spinach Salad

Preparation Time: 10 minutes

Cooking Time: 0 minutes

Servings: 2

Ingredients:

- 2 bunches fresh spinach
- 1 bunch scallions, chopped
- juice of 1 lemon
- 1/4 tbsp. olive oil
- pepper to taste
- optional: rice vinegar to taste

Directions:

1. Wash spinach well. Drain and chop.
2. After a few minutes, squeeze excess water.
3. Add scallions, lemon juice, oil, and pepper.

Nutrition:

- ✓ Calories: 157 kcal
- ✓ Protein: 13.6 g
- ✓ Fat: 6.86 g
- ✓ Carbohydrates: 16.7 g

FISH AND SEAFOOD RECIPES

Lemon-Caper Trout with Caramelized Shallots

Preparation Time: 10 minutes

Cooking Time: 20 minutes

Servings: 2

Ingredients:

- For the Shallots
- 2 shallots, thinly sliced
- 1 teaspoon ghee
- Dash salt
- For the Trout
- 1 tablespoon plus 1 teaspoon ghee, divided
- 2 (4-ounce) trout fillets
- ¼ cup freshly squeezed lemon juice
- 3 tablespoons capers
- ¼ teaspoon salt
- Dash freshly ground black pepper
- 1 lemon, thinly sliced

Directions:

To make the Shallot:

1. In a huge skillet on medium heat, cook the shallots, ghee, and salt for 20 minutes, stirring every 5 minutes, until the shallots have fully wilted and caramelized.

To make the Trout:

2. While the shallots cook, in another large skillet over medium heat, heat 1 teaspoon of ghee.
3. Add the trout fillets. Cook for at least 3 minutes each side, or until the center is flaky. Transfer to a plate and set aside.
4. In the skillet used for the trout, add the lemon juice, capers, salt, and pepper. Bring it to a simmer. Whisk in the remaining 1 tablespoon of ghee. Spoon the sauce over the fish.
5. Garnish the fish with the lemon slices and caramelized shallots before serving.

Nutrition:

- ✓ Calories: 399
- ✓ Total Fat: 22g
- ✓ Saturated Fat: 10g
- ✓ Cholesterol: 46mg
- ✓ Carbohydrates: 17g
- ✓ Fiber: 2g
- ✓ Protein: 21g

Manhattan-Style Salmon Chowder

Preparation Time: 10 minutes

Cooking Time: 15 minutes

Servings: 4

Ingredients:

- ¼ cup Extra Virgin Olive Oil
- 1 Red Bell Pepper, Chopped
- 1 Pound Skinless Salmon. Pin Bones removed, chopped into ½ inch
- 2 (28 oz.) Cans Crushed Tomatoes, 1 Drained, 1 undrained
- 6 cups No salt added chicken broth
- 2 cups diced (1/2 inch) Sweet Potato
- 1 tsp. Onion Powder

- ½ tsp. Sea Salt
- ¼ tsp. Freshly Ground Black Pepper

Directions:

1. Add the red bell pepper and salmon. Cook for at least 5 minutes, occasionally stirring, until the fish is opaque and the bell pepper is soft.
2. Stir in the tomatoes, chicken broth, sweet potatoes, onion powder, salt, and pepper. Place to a simmer then lower the heat to medium. Cook for at least 10 minutes, occasionally stirring, until the sweet potatoes are soft.

Nutrition:

- ✓ Calories: 570
- ✓ Total Fat: 42
- ✓ Total Carbs: 55g
- ✓ Sugar: 24g
- ✓ Fiber: 16g
- ✓ Protein: 41g
- ✓ Sodium: 1,249mg

Roasted Salmon and Asparagus

Preparation Time: 5 minutes

Cooking Time: 15 minutes

Servings: 4

Ingredients:

- 1 pound Asparagus Spears, trimmed
- 2 tbsp. Extra Virgin Olive Oil
- 1 tsp. Sea Salt, divide
- 1½ pound Salmon, cut into 4 fillets
- ⅛ tsp. freshly ground cracked black pepper
- 1 Lemon, zest, and slice

Directions:

1. Preheat the oven to 425°F.
2. Stir the asparagus with the olive oil then put ½ teaspoon of the salt. Place in a single layer in the bottom of a roasting pan.

3. Season the salmon with the pepper and the remaining ½ teaspoon of salt. Put skin-side down on top of the asparagus.
4. Sprinkle the salmon and asparagus with the lemon zest and place the lemon slices over the fish.
5. Roast at the oven for at least 12 to 15 minutes until the flesh is opaque.

Nutrition:

- ✓ Calories: 308
- ✓ Total Fat: 18g
- ✓ Total Carbs: 5g
- ✓ Sugar: 2g
- ✓ Fiber: 2g
- ✓ Protein: 36g
- ✓ Sodium: 545mg

Citrus Salmon on a Bed of Greens

Preparation Time: 10 minutes

Cooking Time: 19 minutes

Servings: 4

Ingredients:

- ¼ cup Extra Virgin Olive Oil, divided
- 1½ pound Salmon
- 1 tsp. Sea Salt, divided
- ½ tsp. Freshly ground black pepper, divided
- 1 Lemon Zest
- 6 cups Swiss Chard, stemmed and chopped
- 3 Garlic cloves, chopped
- 2 Lemon Juice

Directions:

1. In a huge nonstick skillet at medium-high heat, heat 2 tablespoons of the olive oil until it shimmers.
2. Season the salmon with ½ teaspoon of the salt, ¼ teaspoon of the pepper, and the lemon zest. Put the salmon to the skillet, skin-side up, and cook for about 7 minutes until the flesh is opaque. Flip the salmon

and cook for at least 3 to 4 minutes to crisp the skin. Set aside on a plate, cover using aluminum foil.

3. Put back the skillet to the heat, add the remaining 2 tablespoons of olive oil, and heat it until it shimmers.
4. Add the Swiss chard. Cook for about 7 minutes, occasionally stirring, until soft.
5. Add the garlic. Cook for 30 seconds, stirring constantly.
6. Sprinkle in the lemon juice, the remaining ½ teaspoon of salt, and the remaining ¼ teaspoon of pepper. Cook for 2 minutes.
7. Serve the salmon on the Swiss chard.

Nutrition:

- ✓ Calories: 363
- ✓ Total Fat: 25
- ✓ Total Carbs: 3g
- ✓ Sugar: 1g
- ✓ Fiber: 1g
- ✓ Protein: 34g
- ✓ Sodium: 662mg

Orange and Maple-Glazed Salmon

Preparation Time: 15 minutes

Cooking Time: 15 minutes

Servings: 4

Ingredients:

- 2 Orange Juice
- 1 Orange Zest
- ¼ cup Pure maple syrup
- 2 tbsp. Low Sodium Soy Sauce
- 1 tsp. Garlic Powder
- 4 4-6 oz. Salmon Fillet, Pin bones removed

Directions:

1. Preheat the oven to 400°F.
2. In a small, shallow dish, whisk the orange juice and zest, maple syrup, soy sauce, and garlic powder.

3. Put the salmon pieces, flesh-side down, into the dish. Let it marinate for 10 minutes.
4. Transfer the salmon, skin-side up, to a rimmed baking sheet and bake for about 15 minutes until the flesh is opaque.

Nutrition:

- ✓ Calories: 297
- ✓ Total Fat: 11
- ✓ Total Carbs: 18g
- ✓ Sugar: 15g
- ✓ Fiber: 1g
- ✓ Protein: 34g
- ✓ Sodium: 528mg

Salmon Ceviche

Preparation Time: 10 minutes +20 resting time

Cooking Time: 0 minutes

Servings: 4

Ingredients:

- 1 pound Salmon, skinless & boneless, cut into bite-size pieces
- ½ cup Fresh squeezed lime juice
- 2 Tomatoes, diced
- ¼ cup Fresh Cilantro Leaves, chopped
- 1 Jalapeno Pepper, seeded and diced
- 2 tbsp. Extra Virgin Olive Oil
- ½ tsp. Sea Salt

Directions:

1. In a medium bowl, put and stir together the salmon and lime juice. Let it marinate for 20 minutes.
2. Stir in the tomatoes, cilantro, jalapeño, olive oil, and salt.

Nutrition:

- ✓ Calories: 222
- ✓ Total Fat: 14g
- ✓ Total Carbs: 3g
- ✓ Sugar: 2g

✓ Fiber: 1g
✓ Protein: 23g
✓ Sodium: 288mg

Cod with Ginger and Black Beans

Preparation Time: 10 minutes

Cooking Time: 15 minutes

Servings: 4

Ingredients:

- 2 tbsp. Extra Virgin Olive Oil
- 4 (6 oz.) Cod Fillets
- 1 tbsp. Grated fresh ginger
- 1 tsp. Sea Salt, divided
- ¼ tsp. Freshly ground black pepper
- 5 Garlic cloves, minced
- 1 (14 oz.) Can Black Beans, drained
- ¼ cup Fresh Cilantro Leaves, chopped

Directions:

1. In a huge nonstick skillet at medium-high heat, heat the olive oil until it shimmers.
2. Season the cod with the ginger, ½ teaspoon of the salt, and the pepper. Put it in the hot oil then cook for at least 4 minutes per side until the fish is opaque. Take off the cod from the pan and set it aside on a platter, tented with aluminum foil.
3. Put back the skillet to the heat and add the garlic. Cook for 30 seconds, stirring constantly.
4. Stir in the black beans and the rest ½ teaspoon of salt. Cook for 5 minutes, stirring occasionally.
5. Stir in the cilantro and spoon the black beans over the cod.

Nutrition:

- Calories: 419
- Total Fat: 2g
- Total Carbs: 33g
- Sugar: 1g
- Fiber: 8g

- Protein: 50g
- Sodium: 605mg

Rosemary-Lemon Cod

Preparation Time: 5 minutes

Cooking Time: 10 minutes

Servings: 4

Ingredients:

- 2 tbsp. Extra Virgin Olive Oil
- 1½ pound Cod, Skin and Bone Removed, cut into 4 fillets
- 1 tbsp. Fresh Rosemary Leaves, chopped
- ½ tsp. Ground black pepper, or more to taste
- ½ tsp. Sea Salt
- 1 Lemon Juice

Directions:

1. In a huge nonstick skillet at medium-high heat, heat the olive oil until it shimmers.
2. Season the cod with the rosemary, pepper, and salt. Put the fish to the skillet and cook for 3 to 5 minutes per side until opaque.
3. Pour the lemon juice over the cod fillets and cook for 1 minute.

Nutrition:

- Calories: 246
- Total Fat: 9g
- Total Carbs: 1g
- Sugar: 1g
- Fiber: 1g
- Protein: 39g
- Sodium: 370mg

Halibut Curry

Preparation Time: 10 minutes

Cooking Time: 10 minutes

Servings: 4

Ingredients:

- 2 tbsp. Extra Virgin Olive Oil
- 2 tsp. Ground Turmeric
- 2 tsp. Curry Powder
- 1½ pound Halibut, skin, and bones removed, cut into 1 inch pieces
- 4 cups No-salt added chicken broth
- 1 (14 oz.) can Lite coconut milk
- ½ tsp. Sea Salt
- ¼ tsp. Freshly ground black pepper

Directions:

1. In a huge nonstick skillet at medium-high, heat the olive oil until it shimmers.
2. Add the turmeric and curry powder. Cook for 2 minutes, constantly stirring, to bloom the spices.
3. Add the halibut, chicken broth, coconut milk, salt, and pepper. Place to a simmer then lower the heat to medium. Simmer for 6 to 7 minutes, stirring occasionally, until the fish is opaque.

Nutrition:

- ✓ Calories: 429
- ✓ Total Fat: 47g
- ✓ Total Carbs: 5g
- ✓ Sugar: 1g
- ✓ Fiber: 1g
- ✓ Protein: 27g
- ✓ Sodium: 507mg

Baked Tomato Hake

Preparation Time: 10 minutes

Cooking Time: 20-25 minutes

Servings: 4

Ingredients:

- ½ c. tomato sauce
- 1 tbsp. olive oil
- Parsley

- 2 sliced tomatoes
- ½ c. grated cheese
- 4 lbs. de-boned and sliced hake fish
- Salt.

Directions:

1. Preheat the oven to 400 degrees F.
2. Season the fish with salt.
3. In a skillet or saucepan, stir-fry the fish in the olive oil until half-done.
4. Take four foil papers to cover the fish.
5. Shape the foil to resemble containers; add the tomato sauce into each foil container.
6. Add the fish, tomato slices, and top with grated cheese.
7. Bake until you get a golden crust, for approximately 20-25 minutes.
8. Open the packs and top with parsley.

Nutrition:

- ✓ Calories: 265
- ✓ Fat: 15 g
- ✓ Carbs: 18 g
- ✓ Protein: 22 g
- ✓ Sugars: 0.5 g
- ✓ Sodium: 94.6 mg

Salmon and Roasted Peppers

Preparation Time: 5 minutes

Cooking Time: 25 minutes

Servings: 4

Ingredients:

- 1 cup red peppers, cut into strips
- 4 salmon fillets, boneless
- ¼ cup chicken stock
- 2 tablespoons olive oil
- 1 yellow onion, chopped
- 1 tablespoon cilantro, chopped
- Pinch of sea salt
- Pinch black pepper

Directions:

1. Warm a pan with the oil on medium-high heat; add the onion and sauté for 5 minutes.
2. Put the fish and cook for at least 5 minutes on each side.
3. Add the rest of the ingredients, introduce the pan in the oven, and cook at 390 degrees F for 10 minutes.
4. Divide the mix between plates and serve.

Nutrition:

- ✓ Calories 265
- ✓ Fat 7
- ✓ Fiber 5
- ✓ Carbs 15
- ✓ Protein 16

Shrimp and Beets

Preparation Time: 10 minutes

Cooking Time: 10 minutes

Servings: 4

Ingredients:

- 1 pound shrimp, peeled and deveined
- 2 tablespoons avocado oil
- 2 spring onions, chopped
- 2 garlic cloves, minced
- 1 beet, peeled and cubed
- 1 tablespoon lemon juice
- Pinch of sea salt
- Pinch of black pepper
- 1 teaspoon coconut aminos

Directions:

1. Warm a pan with the oil on medium-high heat, add the spring onions and the garlic and sauté for 2 minutes.
2. Add the shrimp and the other ingredients, toss, cook the mix for 8 minutes, divide into bowls and serve.

Nutrition:

- ✓ Calories 281

- ✓ Fat 6
- ✓ Fiber 7
- ✓ Carbs 11
- ✓ Protein 8

Shrimp and Corn

Preparation Time: 5 minutes

Cooking Time: 10 minutes

Servings: 4

Ingredients:

- 1 pound shrimp, peeled and deveined
- 2 garlic cloves, minced
- 1 cup corn
- ½ cup veggie stock
- 1 bunch parsley, chopped
- Juice of 1 lime
- 2 tablespoons olive oil
- Pinch of sea salt
- Pinch of black pepper

Directions:

1. Warm a pan with the oil on medium-high heat, then put the garlic and the corn and sauté for 2 minutes.
2. Add the shrimp and the other ingredients, toss, cook everything for 8 minutes more, divide between plates and serve.

Nutrition:

- ✓ Calories: 343 kcal
- ✓ Protein: 29.12 g
- ✓ Fat: 10.97 g
- ✓ Carbohydrates: 34.25 g

Poached Halibut and Mushrooms

Preparation Time: 5 minutes

Cooking Time: 30 minutes

Servings: 8

Ingredients:

- 1/8 teaspoon sesame oil
- 2 pounds halibut, cut into bite-sized pieces
- 1 teaspoon fresh lemon juice
- ½ teaspoon soy sauce
- 4 cups mushrooms, sliced ¼ cup water
- Salt and pepper to taste ¾ cup green onions

Directions:

1. Place a heavy-bottomed pot on medium-high fire.
2. Add all ingredients and mix well.
3. Cover and bring to a boil. Once boiling, lower fire to a simmer. Cook for 25 minutes.
4. Adjust seasoning to taste.
5. Serve and enjoy.

Nutrition:

- ✓ Calories: 217 Cal
- ✓ Fat 15.8 g
- ✓ Carbs: 1.1 g
- ✓ Protein: 16.5 g
- ✓ Fiber: 0.4 g

Halibut Stir Fry

Preparation Time: 5 minutes

Cooking Time: 20 minutes

Servings: 6

Ingredients:

- 2 pounds halibut fillets
- 2 tbsp. olive oil ½ cup fresh parsley
- 1 onion, sliced 2 stalks celery, chopped
- 2 tablespoons capers
- 4 cloves of garlic minced
- Salt and pepper to taste

Directions:

1. Place a heavy-bottomed pot on high fire and heat for 2 minutes. Add oil and heat for 2 more minutes.

2. Stir in garlic and onions. Sauté for 5 minutes. Add remaining ingredients except for the parsley and stir fry for 10 minutes or until fish is cooked.
3. Adjust seasoning to taste and serve with a sprinkle of parsley.

Nutrition:

- ✓ Calories 331 Cal
- ✓ Fat 26 g
- ✓ Carbs 2 g
- ✓ Protein 22 g
- ✓ Fiber 0.5 g

Steamed Garlic-Dill Halibut

Preparation Time: 5 minutes

Cooking Time: 25 minutes

Servings: 4

Ingredients:

- 1-pound halibut fillet
- 1 lemon, freshly squeezed
- Salt and pepper to taste
- 1 teaspoon garlic powder
- 1 tablespoon dill weed, chopped

Directions:

1. Place a large pot on medium fire and fill up to 1.5-inches of water. Place a trivet inside the pot.
2. In a baking dish that fits inside your large pot, add all ingredients and mix well. Cover dish with foil. Place the dish on top of the trivet inside the pot.
3. Cover pot and steam fish for 15 minutes.
4. Let fish rest for at least 10 minutes before removing from pot.
5. Serve and enjoy.

Nutrition:

- ✓ Calories: 270 Cal
- ✓ Fat: 6.5 g
- ✓ Carbs: 3.9 g
- ✓ Protein: 47.8 g
- ✓ Fiber: 2.1 g

Italian Halibut Chowder

Preparation Time: 5 minutes

Cooking Time: 20 minutes

Servings: 8

Ingredients:

- 2 tablespoons olive oil
- 1 onion, chopped
- 3 stalks of celery, chopped
- 3 cloves of garlic, minced
- 2 ½ pounds halibut steaks, cubed
- 1 red bell pepper, seeded and chopped
- 1 cup tomato juice
- ½ cup apple juice, organic and unsweetened
- ½ teaspoon dried basil
- 1/8 teaspoon dried thyme
- Salt and pepper to taste

Directions:

1. Place a heavy-bottomed pot on medium-high fire and heat pot for 2 minutes. Add oil and heat for a minute.
2. Sauté the onion, celery, and garlic until fragrant.
3. Stir in the halibut steaks and bell pepper. Sauté for 3 minutes.
4. Pour in the rest of the ingredients and mix well.
5. Cover and bring to a boil. Once boiling, lower fire to a simmer and simmer for 10 minutes.
6. Adjust seasoning to taste.
7. Serve and enjoy.

Nutrition:

- ✓ Calories: 318 Cal
- ✓ Fat: 23g
- ✓ Carbs: 6g
- ✓ Protein: 21g
- ✓ Fiber: 1g

Dill Haddock

Preparation Time: 10 minutes

Cooking Time: 30 minutes

Servings: 4

Ingredients:

- 1-pound haddock fillets
- 3 teaspoons veggie stock
- 2 tablespoons lemon juice
- Salt and black pepper to the taste
- 2 tablespoons mayonnaise
- 2 teaspoons chopped dill
- A drizzle of olive oil

Directions:

1. Grease a baking dish with the oil, add the fish, and also add stock mixed with lemon juice, salt, pepper, mayo, and dill. Toss a bit and place in the oven at 350 degrees F to bake for 30 minutes. Divide between plates and serve.
2. Enjoy!

Nutrition:

- ✓ Calories: 214
- ✓ Fat: 12 Cal
- ✓ Fiber: 4 g
- ✓ Carbs: 7 g
- ✓ Protein: 17 g

Honey Crusted Salmon with Pecans

Preparation Time: 20 minutes

Cooking Time: 20 minutes

Servings: 6

Ingredients:

- 3 tablespoons olive oil
- 3 tablespoons mustard
- 5 teaspoons raw honey
- ½ cup chopped pecans
- 6 salmon fillets, boneless
- 3 teaspoons chopped parsley
- Salt and black pepper to the taste

Directions:

1. In a bowl, whisk the mustard with honey and oil. In another bowl, mix the pecans with parsley and stir. Season salmon fillets with salt and pepper, place them on a baking sheet, brush with mustard mixture, top with the pecans mix, and place them in the oven at 400 degrees F to bake for 20 minutes. Divide into plates and serve with a side salad.
2. Enjoy!

Nutrition:

- ✓ Calories 200
- ✓ Fat 10
- ✓ Fiber 5
- ✓ Carbs 12
- ✓ Protein 16

Salmon and Cauliflower

Preparation Time: 10 minutes

Cooking Time: 25 minutes

Servings: 4

Ingredients:

- 2 tablespoons coconut aminos
- 1 cauliflower head, florets separated and chopped
- 4 pieces salmon fillets, skinless
- 1 big red onion, cut into wedges
- 1 tablespoon olive oil
- Pinch of sea salt
- Pinch black pepper

Directions:

1. Put the salmon in a baking dish, put the oil all over, and season with salt and pepper. Place in preheated broiler over medium heat and cook for about 5 minutes. Add coconut aminos, cauliflower, and onion, then place in the oven and bake at 400 degrees F for 15 minutes more. Divide between plates and serve.
2. Enjoy!

Nutrition:

- ✓ Calories 112

- ✓ Fat 5
- ✓ Fiber 3
- ✓ Carbs 8
- ✓ Protein 7

Ginger Salmon and Black Beans

Preparation Time: 10 minutes

Cooking Time: 30 minutes

Servings: 4

Ingredients:

- 1 cup canned black beans, drained
- 2 tablespoons coconut aminos
- ½ cup olive oil
- 1 ½ cup chicken stock
- 6 ounces salmon fillets, boneless
- 2 garlic cloves, minced
- 1 tablespoon fresh grated ginger
- 2 teaspoons white wine vinegar
- ¼ cup grated radishes
- ¼ cup grated carrots
- ¼ cup chopped scallions

Directions:

1. Meanwhile, in a bowl, mix the aminos with half of the oil and whisk. Cut halfway into each salmon fillet, place them in a baking dish and pour the aminos mixture all over. Toss and keep in the fridge for 10 minutes to marinate. Heat a pan with the rest of the oil over medium heat, add garlic, ginger, and black beans. Stir and cook for 3 minutes. Add vinegar and stock, stir, bring to a boil, cook for 10 minutes, and divide between plates. Broil fish for 4 minutes per side over medium-high heat then place a fillet next to the black beans and top with grated scallions, radishes, and carrots.
2. Enjoy!

Nutrition:

- ✓ Calories 200
- ✓ Fat 7
- ✓ Fiber 2
- ✓ Carbs 9
- ✓ Protein 9

Cod Curry

Preparation Time: 10 minutes

Cooking Time: 25 minutes

Servings: 4

Ingredients:

- 4 cod fillets, boneless
- ½ teaspoon mustard seeds
- Salt and black pepper to the taste
- 2 green chilies, chopped
- 1 teaspoon fresh grated ginger
- 1 teaspoon curry powder
- ¼ teaspoon ground cumin
- 4 tablespoons olive oil
- 1 small red onion, chopped
- 1 teaspoon ground turmeric
- ¼ cup chopped parsley
- 1½ cups coconut cream
- 3 garlic cloves, minced

Directions:

1. Heat a pot with half of the oil over medium heat. Add mustard seeds and cook for 2 minutes. Add ginger, onion, garlic, turmeric, curry powder, chilies, and cumin, stir and cook for 10 minutes more. Add coconut milk, salt and pepper then stir. Bring to a boil, cook for 10 minutes and take off the heat. Warm another pan with the rest of the oil over medium heat, add fish, and then cook for 4 minutes. Transfer the fish on top of the curry mix, toss gently then cook for 6 more minutes. Divide between plates, sprinkle the parsley on top and serve.
2. Enjoy!

Nutrition:

- ✓ Calories 210
- ✓ Fat 14
- ✓ Fiber 7
- ✓ Carbs 6
- ✓ Protein 16

Healthy Fish Nacho Bowl

Preparation Time: 13 minutes

Cooking Time: 20 minutes

Servings: 4

Ingredients:

- 500g white fish fillets
- 400g red cabbage
- 3 green shallots
- 1 tablespoon yogurt
- 1 tablespoon olive oil
- 425g can black beans
- 50g gluten-free corn chips
- 200g cherry tomatoes
- 2-3 teaspoons gluten-free chipotle seasoning
- 1 small avocado
- 1/3 cup fresh coriander leaves
- 1 large lime, rind finely grated, juiced

Directions:

1. Combine the fish, stew powder/chipotle flavoring & 2 tsps. oil in a bowl
2. Shred the cabbage in a nourishment processor fitted with the cutting connection. Move to a huge bowl with the tomato, lime skin, dark beans, yogurt, and 2 tbsps. lime juice, 2 shallots, & the rest of the oil. Hurl well to consolidate.
3. Heat a huge non-stick skillet over high warmth. Cook the fish, turning until simply cooked through. Move to a plate.
4. Meanwhile, consolidate the avocado, coriander, remaining shallot & 1 tbsp. remaining lime squeeze in a little bowl.
5. Divide the cabbage blend, fish, guacamole & corn chips among serving bowls. Sprinkle with additional coriander & present with additional lime wedges.

Nutrition:

- ✓ Calories: 388 kcal
- ✓ Protein: 28.17 g
- ✓ Fat: 16.64 g
- ✓ Carbohydrates: 35.72 g

Fish & Chickpea Stew

Preparation Time: 5 minutes

Cooking Time: 10 minutes

Servings: 4

Ingredients:

- 2 cups fish stock
- 1 brown onion
- 400g can tomatoes
- 4 kale leaves
- 500g firm white fish fillets
- Sliced Coles Bakery Stone
- 2 garlic clove
- Finely grated parmesan
- 400g can chickpeas
- 1 carrot, peeled
- Salt & pepper to taste

Directions:

1. Spray a skillet with olive oil shower. Spot over medium-low warmth. Include the carrot & onion & cook, mixing, until delicate & brilliant. Include garlic & cook, blending, until sweet-smelling.
2. Add the chickpeas stock & tomato, & to the onion blend in the skillet. Bring to the bubble. Lessen warmth to medium-low & stew until the blend thickens somewhat.
3. Add the kale & fish to the dish & stew until the fish is simply cooked through. Season.
4. Divide the stew among serving bowls. Sprinkle with parmesan & present with the bread.

Nutrition:

- ✓ Calories: 1447 kcal
- ✓ Protein: 42.1 g
- ✓ Fat: 127.85 g
- ✓ Carbohydrates: 32.4 g

Easy Crunchy Fish Tray Bake

Preparation Time: 10 minutes

Cooking Time: 20 minutes

Servings: 4

Ingredients:

- 600g frozen crumbed whiting fish fillets
- 1/2 small red onion
- 2 x 250g punnets tomatoes

- 2 zucchini
- 180g baby stuffed peppers
- 1 tablespoon parmesan
- 2 teaspoons oregano leaves
- 1 lemon, cut into wedges

Directions:

1. Preheat the stove to 400F. Oil an enormous preparing plate. Spot the fish filets on the readied plate. Disperse the oregano & parmesan over the fish.
2. Add the zucchini, tomatoes & stuffed peppers to the plate. Disperse the onion rings over the top. Season well. Splash with olive oil. Heat until the fish is brilliant & cooked through.
3. Divide the fish & vegetables among plates & present with the rocket & lemon wedges.

Nutrition:

- ✓ Calories: 346 kcal
- ✓ Protein: 3.67 g
- ✓ Fat: 2.8 g
- ✓ Carbohydrates: 81.77 g

Ginger & Chili Sea Bass Fillets

Preparation Time: 5 minutes

Cooking Time: 10 minutes

Servings: 2

Ingredients:

- 2 Sea bass fillet
- 1 tsp. Black pepper
- 1 tbsp. Extra virgin olive oil
- 1 tsp. Ginger, peeled and chopped
- 1 Garlic cloves, thinly slice
- 1 Red chili, deseeded and thinly sliced
- 2 Green onion stemmed, chopped

Directions:

1. Get a skillet and heat the oil on a medium to high heat.
2. Sprinkle black pepper over the Sea Bass and score the fish's skin a few times with a sharp knife.
3. Add the sea bass fillet to the very hot pan with the skin side down.

4. Cook for 5 minutes and turn over.
5. Cook for a further 2 minutes.
6. Remove sea bass from the pan and rest.
7. Put the chili, garlic, and ginger and cook for approximately 2 minutes or until golden.
8. Remove from the heat and add the green onions.
9. Scatter the vegetables over your sea bass to serve.
10. Try with a steamed sweet potato or side salad.

Nutrition:

- ✓ Calories: 306 kcal
- ✓ Protein: 29.92 g
- ✓ Fat: 8.94 g
- ✓ Carbohydrates: 26.59 g

Nut-Crust Tilapia with Kale

Preparation Time: 5 minutes

Cooking Time: 15 minutes

Servings: 2

Ingredients:

- 2 tsp. Extra virgin olive oil
- 2 tbsp. Low-fat hard cheese, grated
- 1/2 cup Roasted and Ground Brazil Nuts/Hazelnuts/Any other hard nut
- 1/2 cup 100% Wholegrain breadcrumbs
- 2 Tilapia Fillet, skinless
- 2 tsp. Whole grain mustard
- 1 Head of kale, chopped
- 1 tbsp. Sesame seeds, lightly toasted
- 1 Garlic clove, minced

Directions:

1. Set the oven to 350°F.
2. Lightly oil a baking sheet with the use of 1 tsp. extra virgin olive oil.
3. Mix in the nuts, breadcrumbs, and cheese in a separate bowl.
4. Spread a thin layer of the mustard over the fish and then dip into the breadcrumb mixture.
5. Transfer to baking dish.

6. Bake for at least 12 minutes, till cooked through.
7. Meanwhile, warm 1 tsp. Oil in a skillet at medium heat temperature then sauté the garlic for 30 seconds, adding in the kale for a further 5 minutes.
8. Mix in the sesame seeds.
9. Serve the fish at once with the kale on the side.

Nutrition:

- ✓ Calories: 475 kcal
- ✓ Protein: 37.14 g
- ✓ Fat: 33.44 g
- ✓ Carbohydrates: 11.08 g

Wasabi Salmon Burgers

Preparation Time: 5 minutes

Cooking Time: 10 minutes

Servings: 1

Ingredients:

- 1/2 tsp. Honey
- 2 tbsp. Reduce-salt soy sauce
- 1 tsp. Wasabi powder
- 1 Beaten free-range egg
- 2 can Wild Salmon, drained
- 2 Scallion, chopped
- 2 tbsp. Coconut Oil
- 1 tbsp. Fresh ginger, minced

Directions:

1. Combine the salmon, egg, ginger, scallions, and 1 tbsp. oil in a bowl, mixing well with your hands to form 4 patties.
2. In a separate bowl, add the wasabi powder and soy sauce with the honey and whisk until blended.
3. Heat 1 tbsp. oil over medium heat in a skillet and cook the patties for 4 minutes each side until firm and browned.
4. Glaze the top of each patty with the wasabi mixture and cook for another 15 seconds before you serve.

5. Serve with your favorite side salad or vegetables for a healthy treat.

Nutrition:

- ✓ Calories: 591 kcal
- ✓ Protein: 63.52 g
- ✓ Fat: 34.3 g
- ✓ Carbohydrates: 3.83 g

Citrus & Herb Sardines

Preparation Time: 5 minutes

Cooking Time: 15 minutes

Servings: 2

Ingredients:

- 10 Sardines, scaled and clean
- 2 Whole Lemon zest
- Handful-Flat leafy parsley, chopped
- 2 Garlic cloves, finely chopped
- 1/2 cup Black Olives (pitted and halves)
- 3 tbsp. Olive oil
- 1 can Tomato, chopped, (optional)
- 1/2 can Chickpeas or Butterbeans, drained and rinsed
- 8 Cherry Tomatoes, halved (optional)
- Pinch of Black Pepper

Directions:

1. In a bowl, add the lemon zest to the chopped parsley (save a pinch for garnishing) and half of the chopped garlic, ready for later.
2. Put a very large skillet on the hob and heat on high.
3. Now add the oil and once very hot, lay the sardines flat on the pan.
4. Sauté for 3 minutes until golden underneath and turn over to fry for another 3 minutes. Place onto a plate to rest.
5. Sauté the remaining garlic (add another splash of oil if you need to) for 1 min until softened. Pour in the tin of chopped tomatoes, mix and let simmer for 4-5 minutes.
6. If you're avoiding tomatoes, just avoid this step and go straight to chickpeas.

7. Tip in the chickpeas or butter beans and fresh tomatoes and stir until heated through.
8. Here's when you add the sardines into the lemon and parsley dressing prepared earlier and add to the pan, cooking for a further 3-4 minutes.
9. Once heated through, serve with a pinch of parsley and remaining lemon zest to garnish.

Nutrition:

- ✓ Calories: 493 kcal
- ✓ Protein: 24.16 g
- ✓ Fat: 35.67 g
- ✓ Carbohydrates: 20.92 g

Spicy Kingfish

Preparation Time: 15 minutes

Cooking Time: 10 minutes

Servings: 2

Ingredients:

- 1 teaspoon dried unsweetened coconut
- 1 teaspoon cumin seeds
- 1 teaspoon fennel seeds
- 1 teaspoon peppercorns
- 10 curry leaves
- ½ teaspoon ground turmeric
- 1½ teaspoons fresh ginger, grated finely
- 1 garlic clove, minced
- Salt, to taste
- 1 tablespoon fresh lime juice
- 4 (4-ounce) kingfish steaks
- 1 tbsp. olive oil
- 1 lime wedge

Directions:

1. Heat a cast-iron skillet on low heat.
2. Add coconut, cumin seeds, fennel seeds, peppercorns, and curry leaves and cook, stirring continuously for about 1 minute.
3. Take off from the heat and cool completely.
4. In a spice grinder, add the spice mixture and turmeric and grind rill powdered finely.

5. Transfer the mixture into a large bowl with ginger, garlic, salt, and lime juice and mix well.
6. Add fish fillets and cat with the mixture evenly.
7. Refrigerate to marinate for about 3 hours.
8. In a huge nonstick skillet, warm oil on medium heat.
9. Put the fish fillets and cook for at least 3-5 minutes per side or till the desired doneness.
10. Transfer onto a paper towel-lined plate to drain.
11. Serve with lime wedges.

Nutrition:

- ✓ Calories: 592 kcal
- ✓ Protein: 67.03 g
- ✓ Fat: 34.55 g
- ✓ Carbohydrates: 4.91 g

Gingered Tilapia

Preparation Time: 15 minutes

Cooking Time: 6 minutes

Servings: 5

Ingredients:

- 2 tablespoons coconut oil
- 5 tilapia fillets
- 3 garlic cloves, minced
- 2 tablespoons unsweetened coconut, shredded
- 4-ounce freshly ground ginger
- 2 tablespoons coconut aminos
- 8 scallions, chopped

Directions:

1. In a huge skillet, melt coconut oil on medium heat.
2. Add tilapia fillets and cook for about 2 minutes.
3. Flip the side and add garlic, coconut, and ginger and cook for about 1 minute.
4. Add coconut aminos and cook for about 1 minute.
5. Add scallion and cook for about 1-2 minutes more.
6. Serve immediately.

Nutrition:

- ✓ Calories: 135
- ✓ Fat: 3g
- ✓ Carbohydrates: 2g
- ✓ Protein: 26g

Haddock with Swiss chard

Preparation Time: 15 minutes

Cooking Time: 10 minutes

Servings: 1

Ingredients:

- 2 tablespoons coconut oil, divided
- 2 minced garlic cloves
- 2 teaspoons fresh ginger, grated finely
- 1 haddock fillet
- Salt, to taste
- Freshly ground black pepper, to taste
- 2 cups Swiss chard, chopped roughly
- 1 teaspoon coconut aminos

Directions:

1. In a skillet, put 1 tablespoon of coconut oil then melt it on medium heat.
2. Add garlic and ginger and sauté for about 1 minute.
3. Add haddock fillet and sprinkle with salt and black pepper.
4. Cook for at least about 3-5 minutes per side or till the desired doneness.
5. Meanwhile, in another skillet, melt remaining coconut oil on medium heat.
6. Add Swiss chard and coconut aminos and cook for about 5-10 minutes.
7. Serve the salmon fillet over Swiss chard.

Nutrition:

- ✓ Calories: 486 kcal
- ✓ Protein: 39.68 g
- ✓ Fat: 34.34 g
- ✓ Carbohydrates: 5.57 g

Coconut Rice with shrimps in Coconut curry

Preparation Time: 10 minutes

Cooking Time: 40 minutes

Servings: 2-3

Ingredients:

- 16 oz. Shrimp (deveined)
- 3 cloves Garlic (chopped)
- 2 Tsp. Curry powder
- ¼ cup Scallions (chopped)
- 15 oz. Coconut milk
- 1 ½ cup Water
- ⅛ cup Cilantro (chopped)
- 2 tbsp.
- Butter
- ½ Lime juice
- 2 tbsp. Ginger (shredded)
- 1 cup Jasmine rice
- Salt and red pepper flakes

Directions:

1. On medium heat, melt 1 tbsp. of butter, then add rice and stir to coat.
2. Pour 1 cup coconut milk and the water and cook for 30 minutes until rice is cooked.
3. Melt butter in a large pan on medium heat, add scallions, garlic, and ginger and leave to cook for 3 minutes.
4. In a separate bowl, mix coconut milk and curry powder
5. After the scallions are cooked, add the shrimps and cook till they are pink.
6. Add the coconut and curry mixture and cook then season accordingly.
7. Remove from heat and serve rice mixed with lime juice and cilantro alongside the shrimps.

Nutrition:

- ✓ Calories: 400 kcal
- ✓ Protein: 40.46 g
- ✓ Fat: 18.01 g
- ✓ Carbohydrates: 29.99 g

Herbed Rockfish

Preparation Time: 10 minutes

Cooking Time: 20 minutes

Servings: 8

Ingredients:

- 1 1/2 pounds rockfish fillets
- 2 egg whites
- 1 1/2 tablespoons nonfat milk
- 1/2 tablespoons canola oil
- 1 cup nonfat plain yogurt
- 1 tablespoon lemon juice
- 1 tablespoon oregano
- 1 tablespoon fresh parsley, chopped
- 1 tablespoon pimento, minced
- 1 teaspoon garlic, minced
- 1 teaspoon ground black pepper
- 6 slices wheat bread, toasted
- 1/4 cup flaxseed, ground fresh
- 1/4 cup extra virgin olive oil
- 1 pint cherry tomatoes, chopped
- 2 fresh lemons, wedges

Directions:

1. Clean rockfish fillets in cold water, remove the skin and remove any bones — Pat dry with paper towels. In a medium-size bowl, combine egg whites, nonfat milk, yogurt, canola oil, and lemon juice — place in a pie pan.
2. Put the next 8 ingredients (oregano-flaxseed) in a food processor until finely ground — place in a separate dish.
3. Heat the olive oil in a pan. First, soak the fillets in the spice mixture, succeeded by the yogurt blend, and then once again in the spice mixture, compressing the crumbs gently into the fish for the final layer.
4. Place the fillets in hot olive oil. When the underneath begins to brown, flip the fillets over, and reduce heat — Cook for a further 15 to 20 minutes.
5. Complete with tomatoes and lemon wedges.

Nutrition:

- ✓ Calories: 178 kcal
- ✓ Protein: 19.62 g
- ✓ Fat: 8.96 g
- ✓ Carbohydrates: 4.73 g

Stuffed Trout

Preparation Time: 20minutes

Cooking Time: 1 hour and 15 minutes

Servings: 4

Ingredients:

- 1 cup chicken broth
- 1/2 cup quinoa
- 2 tablespoons omega-3-rich margarine
- 1 yellow onion, finely dices
- 1 cup (100 g) mushrooms, sliced
- 2 teaspoons dehydrated tarragon
- Salt and pepper
- 1 cup cherry tomatoes, chopped
- 2 tablespoons lemon juice
- 2 tablespoons canola oil
- 2 whole lake trout
- 2 tablespoons flour

Directions:

1. In a pan, place the chicken broth on to simmer. Combine the quinoa, cover, and decrease the heat to low — Cook for 45 to 60 minutes.
2. Preheat oven to 400°F and proceed to line a baking tray with parchment paper.
3. To make the stuffing, melt margarine in a wide pan over medium heat. Sauté the onions and mushrooms till tender. Season by including tarragon, and salt and pepper. Combine cherry tomatoes and sauté 1 to 2 minutes further, mixing continually. Take off the heat and combine with cooked quinoa. Add in lemon juice and stir.
4. Spray the canola oil covering the trout. In a bowl, blend together flour, salt, and pepper. Glaze the interior and exterior of the trout with the flour batter. Stuff the trout with the stuffing blend.
5. Cook uncovered for 10 minutes per inch of trout.

Nutrition:

- ✓ Calories: 342 kcal
- ✓ Protein: 18.76 g
- ✓ Fat: 19.1 g
- ✓ Carbohydrates: 24.38 g

Thai Chowder

Preparation Time: 10 minutes

Cooking Time: 20 minutes

Servings: 6

Ingredients:

- 3 cups 98 % fat-free chicken broth
- 10 small red potatoes, diced
- 3 cobs fresh sweet corn
- 3/4 cup coconut milk
- 1/2 teaspoon fresh ginger, diced
- 1 teaspoon dried lemongrass
- 1 teaspoon green curry paste
- 1/2 cup cabbage, chopped
- Four 5-ounce tilapia fillets
- 2 tablespoons fish sauce
- 3/4 cup fresh shrimp, cleaned, with tails on
- 3/4 cup bay scallops
- 3/4 cup cilantro, chopped

Directions:

1. In a saucepan, boil chicken stock at high heat until it reaches a simmer. Decrease temperature and add the cabbage, ginger, coconut milk, lemongrass, sweet corn, and lemongrass, curry paste, and potatoes — cover and cook for 15 minutes.
2. Firstly, combine fish fillets and fish sauce, and cook for 6 minutes. Secondly, add the shrimp, and cook for a further 2 to 3 minutes. Finally, add the scallops and cook until scallops are opaque in color.
3. Serve with cilantro.

Nutrition:

- ✓ Calories: 761 kcal
- ✓ Protein: 33.25 g
- ✓ Fat: 5.34 g
- ✓ Carbohydrates: 150.45 g

Seared Ahi Tuna

Preparation Time: 10 minutes

Cooking Time: 15 minutes

Servings: 2

Ingredients:

- 2 (4-ounces each) ahi tuna steaks (3/4-inch thick)

- 2 tbsp. dark sesame oil
- 2 tbsp. soy sauce
- 1 tbsp. of grated fresh ginger
- 1 clove garlic, minced
- 1 green onion (scallion) thinly sliced, reserve a few slices for garnish
- 1 tsp. lime juice

Directions:

1. Begin by preparing the marinade. In a small bowl, put together the sesame oil, soy sauce, fresh ginger, minced garlic, green onion, and lime juice. Mix well.
2. Place tuna steaks into a sealable Ziploc freezer bag and pour marinade over the top of the tuna. Seal bag and shake or massage with hands to coat tuna steaks well with marinade. Bring the bag in a bowl, in case of breaks, and place tuna in the refrigerator to marinate for at least 10 minutes.
3. Place a large non-stick skillet over medium-high to high heat. Let the pan heat for 2 minutes, when hot, remove tuna steaks from the marinade and lay them in the pan to sear for 1-1½ minutes on each side.
4. Remove tuna steaks from pan and cut into ¼-inch thick slices. Garnish with a sprinkle of sliced green onion. Serve immediately.

Nutrition:

- ✓ Calories: 213 kcal
- ✓ Protein: 4.5 g
- ✓ Fat: 19.55 g
- ✓ Carbohydrates: 5.2 g

Quick Shrimp Moqueca

Preparation Time: 10 minutes

Cooking Time: 10 minutes

Servings: 4

Ingredients:

- 600g Shrimp Peeled and Clean
- Salt to taste
- Juice of 2 lemons
- Braised olive oil
- 2 chopped purple onions

- 4 cloves garlic, minced
- 3 chopped tomatoes
- 1 chopped red pepper
- 1 chopped yellow pepper
- 1 cup tomato passata
- 200ml of coconut milk
- 2 finger peppers
- 2 tablespoons palm oil
- Chopped cilantro to taste

Directions:

1. In a container, arrange shrimp, season with salt and lemon juice and set aside.
2. In a hot pan, arrange olive oil and sauté onion and garlic.
3. Add the chopped tomatoes and sauté well.
4. Add the peppers and the tomato passata. Let it cook for a few minutes.
5. Add coconut milk, mix well.
6. Add the shrimp to the sauce.
7. Finally, add the finger pepper, palm oil, and chopped coriander.
8. Serve with rice and crumbs.

Nutrition:

- ✓ Calories: 426 kcal
- ✓ Protein: 46.15 g
- ✓ Fat: 15.46 g
- ✓ Carbohydrates: 26.26 g

Souvlaki Spiced Salmon Bowls

Preparation Time: 10 minutes

Cooking Time: 20 minutes

Servings: 4

Ingredients:

For the Salmon:

- ¼ cup good-quality olive oil
- Juice of 1 lemon
- 2 tablespoons chopped fresh oregano
- 1 tablespoon minced garlic
- 1 tablespoon balsamic vinegar
- 1 tablespoon smoked sweet paprika
- ½ teaspoon sea salt
- ¼ teaspoon freshly ground black pepper
- 4 (4-ounce) salmon fillets

Directions:

1. To make the Salmon:
2. Marinate the fish. In a medium bowl, put and mix the olive oil, lemon juice, oregano, garlic, vinegar, paprika, salt, and pepper. Put the salmon and turn to coat it well with the marinade. Cover the bowl and let the salmon sit marinating for 15 to 20 minutes.
3. Grill the fish. Preheat the grill to medium-high heat and grill the fish until just cooked through, 4 to 5 minutes per side. Set the fish aside on a plate.

For the Bowls:

- 2 tablespoons good-quality olive oil
- 1 red bell pepper, cut into strips
- 1 yellow bell pepper, cut into strips
- 1 zucchini, cut into ½-inch strips lengthwise
- 1 cucumber, diced
- 1 large tomato, chopped
- ½ cup sliced Kalamata olives
- 6 ounces feta cheese, crumbled
- ½ cup sour cream

Directions:

To make the Bowls:

1.
   Grill the vegetables. In a medium bowl, put the oil, red and yellow bell peppers, and zucchini. Grill the vegetables, turning once, until they are lightly charred and soft, about 3 minutes per side.
2. Assemble and serve. Divide the grilled vegetables between four bowls. Top each bowl with cucumber, tomato, olives, feta cheese, and the sour cream. Put 1 salmon fillet on top of every bowl and serve immediately.

Nutrition:

- ✓ Calories: 553
- ✓ Total fat: 44g
- ✓ Total carbs: 10g
- ✓ Fiber: 3g;
- ✓ Net carbs: 7g
- ✓ Sodium: 531mg

- ✓ Protein: 30g

Prosciutto-Wrapped Haddock

Preparation Time: 10 minutes

Cooking Time: 15 minutes

Servings: 4

Ingredients:

- 4 (4-ounce) haddock fillets, about 1 inch thick
- Sea salt, for seasoning
- Freshly ground black pepper, for seasoning
- 4 slices prosciutto (2 ounces)
- 3 tablespoons garlic-infused olive oil
- Juice and zest of 1 lemon

Directions:

1. Preheat the oven. Set the oven temperature to 350°F. Line a baking sheet with parchment paper.
2. Prepare the fish. Pat the fish dry using paper towels then spice it lightly on both sides with salt and pepper. Wrap the prosciutto around the fish tightly but carefully so it doesn't rip.
3. Bake the fish. Bring the fish on the baking sheet and drizzle it with the olive oil. Bake for 15 to 17 minutes until the fish flakes easily with a fork.
4. Serve. Divide the fish between four plates and top with the lemon zest and a drizzle of lemon juice.

Nutrition:

- ✓ Calories: 282
- ✓ Total fat: 18g
- ✓ Total carbs: 1g
- ✓ Fiber: 0g;
- ✓ Net carbs: 1g
- ✓ Sodium: 76mg
- ✓ Protein: 29g

Grilled Salmon with Caponata

Preparation Time: 15 minutes

Cooking Time: 20 minutes

Servings: 4

Ingredients:

- ¼ cup good-quality olive oil, divided
- 1 onion, chopped
- 2 celery stalks, chopped
- 1 tablespoon minced garlic
- 2 tomatoes, chopped
- ½ cup chopped marinated artichoke hearts
- ¼ cup pitted green olives, chopped
- ¼ cup cider vinegar
- 2 tablespoons white wine
- 2 tablespoons chopped pecans
- 4 (4-ounce) salmon fillets
- Freshly ground black pepper, for seasoning
- 2 tablespoons chopped fresh basil

Direction:

1. Make the caponata. In a large skillet at medium heat, warm 3 tablespoons of the olive oil.
2. Add the onion, celery, garlic, and sauté until they have softened, about 4 minutes. Stir in the tomatoes, artichoke hearts, olives, vinegar, white wine, and pecans. Place the mixture to a boil, then reduce the heat to low and simmer until the liquid has reduced, 6 to 7 minutes. Take off the skillet from the heat and set it aside.
3. Grill the fish. Preheat a grill to medium-high heat. Pat the fish dry using paper towels then rub it with the remaining 1 tablespoon of olive oil and season lightly with black pepper. Grill the salmon, turning once, until it is just cooked through, about 8 minutes total.
4. Serve. Divide the salmon between four plates, top with a generous scoop of the caponata, and serve immediately with fresh basil.

Nutrition:

- ✓ Calories: 348
- ✓ Total fat: 25g
- ✓ Total carbs: 7g
- ✓ Fiber: 3g
- ✓ Net carbs: 4g
- ✓ Sodium: 128mg

- ✓ Protein: 24g

Herbed Coconut Milk Steamed Mussels

Preparation Time: 10 minutes

Cooking Time: 15 minutes

Servings: 4

Ingredients:

- 2 tablespoons coconut oil
- ½ sweet onion, chopped
- 2 teaspoons minced garlic
- 1 teaspoon grated fresh ginger
- ½ teaspoon turmeric
- 1 cup coconut milk
- Juice of 1 lime
- 1½ pounds fresh mussels, scrubbed and debearded
- 1 scallion, finely chopped
- 2 tablespoons chopped fresh cilantro
- 1 tablespoon chopped fresh thyme

Directions:

1. Sauté the aromatics. In a huge skillet, warm the coconut oil. Add the onion, garlic, ginger, and turmeric and sauté until they have softened, about 3 minutes.
2. Add the liquid. Mix in the coconut milk, lime juice then bring the mixture to a boil.
3. Steam the mussels. Put the mussels to the skillet, cover, and steam until the shells are open, about 10 minutes. Take the skillet off the heat and throw out any unopened mussels.
4. Add the herbs. Stir in the scallion, cilantro, and thyme.
5. Divide the mussels and the sauce into 4 bowls and serve them immediately.

Nutrition:

- ✓ Calories: 319
- ✓ Total fat: 23g
- ✓ Total carbs: 8g
- ✓ Fiber: 2g;
- ✓ Net carbs: 6g
- ✓ Sodium: 395mg

✓ Protein: 23g

Basil Halibut Red Pepper Packets

Preparation Time: 10 minutes

Cooking Time: 20 minutes

Servings: 4

Ingredients:

- 2 cups cauliflower florets
- 1 cup roasted red pepper strips
- ½ cup sliced sun-dried tomatoes
- 4 (4-ounce) halibut fillets
- ¼ cup chopped fresh basil
- Juice of 1 lemon
- ¼ cup good-quality olive oil
- Sea salt, for seasoning
- Freshly ground black pepper, for seasoning

Directions:

1. Preheat the oven. Set the oven temperature to 400°F. Cut into four (12-inch) square pieces of aluminum foil. Have a baking sheet ready.
2. Make the packets. Divide the cauliflower, red pepper strips, and sun-dried tomato between the four pieces of foil, placing the vegetables in the middle of each piece.
3. Top each pile with 1 halibut fillet, and top each fillet with equal amounts of the basil, lemon juice, and olive oil. Fold and crimp the foil to form sealed packets of fish and vegetables and place them on the baking sheet.
4. Bake the packets for about 20 minutes, until the fish flakes with a fork. Be careful of the steam when you open the packet!
5. Transfer the vegetables and halibut to four plates, season with salt and pepper, and serve immediately.

Nutrition:

- ✓ Calories: 294
- ✓ Total fat: 18g
- ✓ Total carbs: 8g
- ✓ Fiber: 3g
- ✓ Net carbs: 5g
- ✓ Sodium: 114mg

✓ Protein: 25g

Oven-Baked Sole Fillets

Preparation Time: 10 minutes

Cooking Time: 20 minutes

Servings: 4

Ingredients:

- 2 tablespoons olive oil
- 1/2 tablespoon Dijon mustard
- 1 teaspoon garlic paste
- 1/2 tablespoon fresh ginger, minced
- 1/2 teaspoon porcini powder
- Salt and ground black pepper, to taste
- 1/2 teaspoon paprika
- 4 sole fillets
- 1/4 cup fresh parsley, chopped

Directions:

1. Combine the oil, Dijon mustard, garlic paste, ginger, porcini powder, salt, black pepper, and paprika.
2. Rub this mixture all over sole fillets. Place the sole fillets in a lightly oiled baking pan.
3. Bake in the preheated oven at 400 degrees F for about 20 minutes

Nutrition:

- ✓ 195 Calories
- ✓ 8.2g Fat
- ✓ 0.5g Carbs
- ✓ 28.7g Protein
- ✓ 0.6g Fiber

Keto Oodles with White Clam Sauce

Preparation Time: 10 minutes

Cooking Time: 10 minutes

Servings: 4

Ingredients:

- 2 pounds small clams
- 8 cups zucchini noodles
- 1/2 cup dry white wine
- 1/4 cup butter
- 1/4 cup fresh parsley (chopped)
- 2 tablespoons lemon juice

- 2 tablespoons olive oil
- 1 tablespoon garlic (minced)
- 1 teaspoon kosher salt
- 1 teaspoon lemon zest (grated)
- 1/4 teaspoon black pepper (ground)

Directions:

1. In a pan at medium heat, place the olive oil, butter, pepper, and salt. Stir to melt the butter.
2. Put in the garlic. Sautee the garlic until fragrant for at least 2 minutes
3. Set in the lemon juice and wine. Cook for at least 2 minutes, until the liquid is slightly reduced
4. Put in the clams. Cook the clams until they are all opened (about 3 minutes). Discard any clam that does not open after 3 minutes.
5. Remove the pan from the heat. Put in the zucchini noodles. Toss the mixture to combine well. Let the noodles rest for a couple of minutes to soften them.
6. Put in the lemon zest and parsley. Stir. Serve.

Nutrition:

- ✓ Calories: 311
- ✓ Carbs: 9 g
- ✓ Fats: 19 g
- ✓ Proteins: 13 g
- ✓ Fiber: 2 g

Fried Codfish with Almonds

Preparation Time: 8 minutes

Cooking Time: 18 minutes

Servings: 3

Ingredients:

- 16 oz. codfish fillet
- 3 oz. chopped almonds
- ½ tsp. chili pepper
- 1 egg
- 1 tbsp. ghee butter
- 1 tsp. psyllium
- 3 oz. cream
- 3 tbsp. keto mayo
- 1 tbsp. chopped fresh dill

- 1 tsp. minced garlic
- ½ tsp. onion powder
- Salt and pepper to taste

Directions:

1. In a small mixing bowl, combine the psyllium, onion powder, chili, and almonds
2. Beat the eggs in another bowl, mix well
3. Warm the butter in a skillet at medium heat.
4. Cut the fillet into 3 slices
5. Dip into the egg mixture, then into almonds and spices
6. Fry in the skillet for about 7 minutes each side
7. Meanwhile, in another bowl combine the cream, garlic, dill, and salt, stir well
8. Serve the fish with this sauce

Nutrition:

- ✓ Carbs: 4, 9 g
- ✓ Fats: 63 g
- ✓ Protein: 33, 6 g
- ✓ Calories: 709

Salmon Balls

Preparation Time: 5 minutes

Cooking Time: 13 minutes

Servings: 2

Ingredients:

- 1 can of tuna
- 2 tbsp. keto mayo
- 1 avocado
- 1 egg
- 1 garlic clove
- ½ cup heavy cream
- 3 tbsp. coconut oil
- ½ tsp. ginger powder
- ½ tsp. paprika
- ½ tsp. dried cilantro
- 2 tbsp. lemon juice
- 2 tbsp. water
- Salt and ground black pepper to taste

Directions:

1. Drain the salmon, chop it

2. Mince the garlic clove, peel the avocado
3. In a bowl, combine the fish, mayo, egg, and garlic, season with salt, paprika, and ginger, mix well
4. Make 4 balls of it
5. Warm the oil in a skillet at medium heat
6. Put the balls and fry for 4-6 minutes each side
7. Meanwhile, put the heavy cream, avocado, cilantro, lemon juice, and 1 tablespoon of oil in a blender. Pulse well
8. Serve the balls with the sauce

Nutrition:

- ✓ Carbs: 3, 9 g
- ✓ Fats: 50 g
- ✓ Protein: 20, 1 g
- ✓ Calories: 555

Codfish Sticks

Preparation Time: 8 minutes

Cooking Time: 15 minutes

Servings: 2

Ingredients:

- 9 oz. codfish fillet
- 2 eggs
- 2 tbsp. ghee butter
- 2 tbsp. coconut flour
- ½ tsp. paprika
- Salt and pepper to taste

Directions:

1. Slice the fish into sticks
2. In a bowl, put and mix the eggs, flour, paprika, pepper, and salt
3. Warm the butter in a skillet at medium heat.
4. Dip each fish slice into the spice mixture
5. Fry in the skillet over low heat for 4-5 minutes per side

Nutrition:

- ✓ Carbs: 1, 5 g
- ✓ Fat: 31 g
- ✓ Protein: 22, 5 g
- ✓ Calories: 329

Lemony Trout

Preparation Time: 10 minutes

Cooking Time: 20 minutes

Servings: 2

Ingredients:

- 5 tbsp. ghee butter
- 5 oz. trout fillets
- 2 garlic cloves
- 1 tsp. rosemary
- 1 lemon
- 2 tbsp. capers
- Salt and pepper to taste

Directions:

1. Preheat the oven to 400F
2. Peel the lemon, mince the garlic cloves and chop the capers
3. Season the trout fillets with salt, rosemary, and pepper
4. Grease a baking dish with the oil and place the fish onto it
5. Warm the butter in a skillet over medium heat
6. Add the garlic and cook for 4-5 minutes until golden
7. Remove from the heat, add the lemon zest and 2 tablespoons of lemon juice, stir well
8. Pour the lemon-butter sauce over the fish and top with the capers
9. Bake for 14-15 minutes. Serve hot

Nutrition:

- ✓ Carbs: 3, 1 g
- ✓ Fat: 25 g
- ✓ Protein: 15, 8 g
- ✓ Calories: 302

Quick Fish Bowl

Preparation Time: 11 minutes

Cooking Time: 15 minutes

Servings: 2

Ingredients:

- 2 tilapia fillets
- 1 tbsp. olive oil

- 1 avocado
- 1 tbsp. ghee butter
- 1 tbsp. cumin powder
- 1 tbsp. paprika
- 2 cups coleslaw cabbage, chopped
- 1 tbsp. salsa sauce
- Himalayan rock salt, to taste
- Black pepper to taste

Directions:

1. Preheat the oven to 425F. Line a baking sheet with the foil
2. Mash the avocado
3. Brush the tilapia fillets using olive oil, season with salt and spices
4. Place the fish onto the baking sheet, greased with the ghee butter
5. Bake for 15 minutes, then remove the fish from the heat and let it cool for 5 minutes
6. In a bowl, combine the coleslaw cabbage and the salsa sauce, toss gently
7. Add the mashed avocado, season with salt and pepper
8. Slice the fish and add to the bowl
9. Bake for 14-15 minutes. Serve hot

Nutrition:

- ✓ Carbs: 5, 2 g
- ✓ Fat: 24, 5 g
- ✓ Protein: 16, 1 g
- ✓ Calories: 321

Tender Creamy Scallops

Preparation Time: 15 minutes

Cooking Time: 21 minutes

Servings: 2

Ingredients:

- 8 fresh sea scallops
- 4 bacon slices
- ½ cup grated parmesan cheese
- 1 cup heavy cream
- 2 tbsp. ghee butter
- Salt and black pepper to taste

Directions:

1. Heat the butter in a skillet at medium-high heat
2. Add the bacon and cook for 4-5 minutes each side (till crispy)
3. Moved to a paper towel to remove the excess fat
4. Lower the heat to medium, sprinkle with more butter. Put the heavy cream and parmesan cheese, season with salt and pepper
5. Reduce the heat to low and cook for 8-10 minutes, constantly stirring, until the sauce thickens
6. In another skillet, heat the ghee butter over medium-high heat
7. Add the scallops to the skillet, season with salt and pepper. Cook for 2 minutes per side until golden
8. Transfer the scallops to a paper towel
9. Top with the sauce and crumbled bacon

Nutrition:

- ✓ Carbs: 11 g
- ✓ Fat: 72, 5 g
- ✓ Protein: 24 g
- ✓ Calories: 765

Salmon Cakes

Preparation Time: 10 minutes

Cooking Time: 10 minutes

Servings: 2

Ingredients:

- 6 oz. canned salmon
- 1 large egg
- 2 tbsp. pork rinds
- 3 tbsp. keto mayo
- 1 tbsp. ghee butter
- 1 tbsp. Dijon mustard
- Salt and ground black pepper to taste

Directions:

1. In a bowl, combine the salmon (drained), pork rinds, egg, and half of the mayo, season with salt and pepper. Mix well

2. With the salmon mixture, form the cakes
3. Heat the ghee butter in a skillet over medium-high heat
4. Place the salmon cakes in the skillet and cook for about 3 minutes per side. Moved to a paper towel to get rid of excess fat
5. In a small bowl, combine the remaining half of mayo and the Dijon mustard, mix well
6. Serve the salmon cakes with the mayo-mustard sauce

Nutrition:

- ✓ Carbs: 1, 2 g
- ✓ Fat: 31 g
- ✓ Protein: 24, 2 g
- ✓ Calories: 370

Salmon with Mustard Cream

Preparation Time: 10 minutes

Cooking Time: 12 minutes

Servings: 2

Ingredients:

- 2 salmon fillets
- ¼ cup keto mayo
- 1 tbsp. Dijon mustard
- 2 tbsp. fresh cilantro, minced
- 2 tbsp. ghee butter
- ½ tsp. garlic powder
- Salt and pepper to taste

Directions:

1. Preheat the oven to 450F. Grease a baking dish with the ghee butter
2. Season the salmon with salt and pepper and put in the baking dish
3. In a mixing bowl, put and combine the Dijon mustard, mayo, parsley, and garlic powder. Stir well
4. Top the salmon fillets with the mustard sauce
5. Bake for 10 minutes

Nutrition:

- ✓ Carbs: 2 g
- ✓ Fat: 41, 5 g
- ✓ Protein: 32, 9 g

- ✓ Calories: 505

Tuna Steaks with Shirataki Noodles

Preparation Time: 10 minutes

Cooking Time: 20 minutes

Servings: 4

Ingredients:

- 1 pack (7 oz.) miracle noodle angel hair
- 3 cups water
- 1 red bell pepper, seeded and halved
- 4 tuna steaks
- Salt and black pepper to taste
- Olive oil for brushing
- 2 tablespoons pickled ginger
- 2 tablespoons chopped cilantro

Directions:

1. Cook the shirataki rice based on the package instructions: In a colander, rinse the shirataki noodles with running cold water.
2. Place a pot of salted water to a boil; blanch the noodles for 2 minutes.
3. Drain and moved to a dry skillet over medium heat.
4. Dry roast for a few minutes until opaque.
5. Grease a grill's grate using a cooking spray and preheat on medium heat. Spice the red bell pepper and tuna with salt and black pepper, brush with olive oil, and grill covered.
6. Cook both for at least 3 minutes on each side. Moved to a plate to cool. Dice bell pepper with a knife.
7. Arrange the noodles, tuna, and bell pepper into the serving plate.
8. Top with pickled ginger and garnish with cilantro.
9. Serve with roasted sesame sauce.

Nutrition:

- ✓ Calories: 310
- ✓ Fat: 18.2g
- ✓ Net Carbs: 2g
- ✓ Protein: 22g

Tilapia with Parmesan Bark

Preparation Time: 4 minutes

Cooking Time: 12 minutes

Servings: 4

Ingredients:

- ¾ cup freshly grated Parmesan cheese
- 2 teaspoons pepper
- 1 tablespoon chopped parsley
- 4 tilapia fillets (4 us)
- Lemon cut into pieces

Directions:

1. Set the oven to 400° F. Mix cheese in a shallow dish with pepper and parsley and season with salt and pepper.
2. Mix the fish in the cheese with olive oil and flirt. Place on a baking sheet with foil and bake for 10 to 12 minutes until the fish in the thickest part is opaque.
3. Serve the lemon slices with the fish.

Nutrition:

- ✓ Calories: 210
- ✓ Fat: 9.3g
- ✓ Net Carbs: 1.3g
- ✓ Protein: 28.9g

Blackened Fish Tacos with Slaw

Preparation Time: 14 minutes

Cooking Time: 6 minutes

Servings: 4

Ingredients:

- 1 tablespoon olive oil
- 1 teaspoon chili powder
- 2 tilapia fillets
- 1 teaspoon paprika
- 4 low carb tortillas

Slaw:

- ½ cup red cabbage, shredded
- 1 tablespoon lemon juice
- 1 teaspoon apple cider vinegar
- 1 tablespoon olive oil

- Salt and black pepper to taste

Directions:

1. Season the tilapia with chili powder and paprika. Heat the vegetable oil during a skillet over medium heat.
2. Add tilapia and cook until blackened, about 3 minutes per side. Cut into strips. Divide the tilapia between the tortillas. Blend all the slaw ingredients in a bowl and top the fish to serve.

Nutrition:

- ✓ Calories: 268
- ✓ Fat: 20g
- ✓ Net Carbs: 3.5g
- ✓ Protein: 13.8g

AIR FRYER (BONUS)

Air Fryer Chicken Tacos

Time for Preparation: Ten min.

Time for Cooking: Twenty min.

Servings: Two-Four servings

Ingredients:

- ✓ 1 lb. of boneless, skinless, thinly cut chicken breasts.
- ✓ olive oil 1 tbsp.
- ✓ Taco seasoning, 1 tbsp.
- ✓ Garlic powder 12 tsp.
- ✓ onion powder 1/8 teaspoon.
- ✓ 12 tsp. salt
- ✓ Black pepper, 1/4 tsp.
- ✓ 6 to 8 tacos
- ✓ Various toppings (such as sour cream, shredded lettuce, chopped tomatoes, and shredded cheese).

Directions:

1. The air fryer should be set at 375 degrees.
2. To thoroughly coat the chicken, combine it with the olive oil, taco seasoning, black pepper, onion powder, garlic powder, and salt in a bowl.
3. Arrange the chicken in a single row in the air fryer basket.
4. After 10 minutes of cooking, flip the chicken strips. Cook the chicken for a further five to seven min, or until it is cooked crispy and thoroughly.
5. Warm the taco shells in the oven or microwave while the chicken cooks.

6. 6. To create the tacos, put the chicken strips in the taco shells and a topping of your choice.

Nutrition:

- ✓ Calories: 328
- ✓ Fat: 11.6 grams.
- ✓ Fiber: 2.9g
- ✓ Protein: 34.3g
- ✓ Carbohydrates: 21.3g

Air Fryer Tofu Stir Fry

Time for Preparation: fifteen min.

Time for Cooking: twenty min.

Servings: Two-Four

Ingredients:

- 1 block (14 oz.) of pressed, drained, and firm tofu
- corn flour, two teaspoons
- 1/4 tsp. of black pepper and half tsp. of salt.
- a quarter-teaspoon of garlic powder
- Paprika, 1/8 teaspoon
- Vegetable oil, 1 tbsp.
- 2 cups of mixed veggies (such as broccoli, carrots, and snap peas), 1 bell pepper, 1 cup chopped onion.
- Soy sauce, 1/4 cup.
- Honey, two tsp.
- a teaspoon of rice vinegar
- 1/8 teaspoon powdered ginger
- A quarter-teaspoon of red pepper flakes
- Corn flour, one tbsp.
- 14 cup of water
- Brown rice two cups, cooked

Directions:

1. The air fryer should be turned on and heated to 400°F.
2. Separate the tofu into small pieces.
3. Combine cornflour, salt, garlic powder, black pepper, and paprika in a small basin.
4. Add the tofu and thoroughly combine with the cornflour mixture.
5. Place the tofu, touching it not at all, in the air fryer basket after spraying it with cooking spray. Spray the tofu with cooking spray.
6. Cook the tofu for a further ten min, or until it becomes golden, after flipping it over.
7. Add the vegetable oil to a large pan and heat it to medium-high. Cook the tofu at this point.
8. Include the onions, peppers, and mixed veggies in the pan and simmer for 5-7 min, or up to it get softened.
9. In a small bowl, combine the rice vinegar, honey, soy sauce, ginger powder, and red pepper flakes. Separately, combine the corn flour and water in a small basin.
10. As you toss the vegetables, pour the sauce over them.
11. Stir thoroughly after adding the cooked tofu to the saucepan.
12. Keep the sauce simmering for a further two to three min, or until the tofu and vegetables are warm.
13. Serve the stir fry over brown rice.

Nutrition:

- ✓ Calories: 329

- ✓ Sodium: 1334mg
- ✓ Protein: 15g
- ✓ Carbohydrates: 49g
- ✓ Fat: 9g
- ✓ Fiber: 7g
- ✓ Sugar: 17g

Air Fryer Breakfast Burritos

Time for Preparation: 15 mints.

Time for Cooking: 10 mints.

Servings: 2-4

Ingredients:

- Four large eggs
- One tbsp. butter
- Black pepper 1/4 tsp.
- Salt 1/4 tsp.
- Milk 1/4 cup.
- 4 flour tortillas
- 1/4 cup chopped fresh cilantro.
- 1/4 cup diced bell pepper.
- 1/4 cup diced onions.
- 1/4 cup diced tomatoes.
- Shredded cheddar cheese half cup.
- Sour cream and Salsa for serving (optional)

Directions:

1. Set your air fryer's temperature to 400°F (200°C).
2. Combine the eggs, black pepper, salt, and milk in a bowl.
3. Heat the butter in a nonstick pan over a moderate flame.
4. Include the egg mixture and keep stirring until the eggs are fully cooked.
5. Spread 2 tablespoons of shredded cheddar cheese in the tortilla's centre after setting it on a level surface.
6. Top with a fourth of the diced tomatoes, onion, bell pepper, cilantro, and scrambled eggs.
7. To assemble a burrito, fold the tortilla's edges inside and roll it up from the bottom up.
8. Carry out with the remaining tortillas and components.
9. Arrange the burritos in the basket of air fryer seam-side down and gently coat with cooking spray.
10. To make the tortillas crispy and golden, air fried the burritos for 8 to 10 minutes.
11. Add salsa and sour cream to the top.

Nutrition:

- ✓ Calories: 365
- ✓ Sugar: 3g
- ✓ Dietary Fiber: 2g
- ✓ Total Carbohydrate: 25g
- ✓ Sodium: 605mg
- ✓ Cholesterol: 241mg
- ✓ Saturated Fat: 10g
- ✓ Total Fat: 22g
- ✓ Protein: 17g
- ✓ Total Carbohydrate: 25g

Air Fryer Mushroom Risotto

Time for Preparation: Ten min.

Time for Cooking: 20 min.

Servings: 2-4

Ingredients:

- Diced onion 1/4 cup.

- Half cup chopped mushrooms.
- Arborio rice one cup.
- Olive oil two tbsp.
- Three cups chicken or vegetable broth.
- White wine 1/4 cup.
- Minced garlic two cloves.
- Fresh parsley, chopped, as a garnish (optional).
- To taste, add salt and pepper.
- Grated Parmesan cheese 1/4 cup.

Directions:

1. Set the air fryer to 200 °C.
2. Mix rice and mushrooms in a bowl.
3. Place rice and mushrooms in air fryer basket and sauté for five mints or until lightly browned.
4. 4. In another container, mix the onions and garlic. Add the onion-garlic mixture to the air fryer basket and bake for five min at a time till it's lightly browned.
5. In a bowl, combine white wine and chicken or vegetable stock.
6. Add the wine and stock combination to the basket of air fryer with the rice mixture.
7. Air fried the rice for 10 to 15 minutes, tossing every 5 min, or till the liquid is entirely absorbed. Sprinkle with olive oil, and then combine with pepper, salt, and parmesan cheese.
8. Garnish with fresh parsley if desired.

Nutrition:

- ✓ Calories: 293
- ✓ Protein: 7g
- ✓ Total Fat: 9g
- ✓ Dietary Fiber: 1g
- ✓ Total Carbohydrate: 43g
- ✓ Sodium: 921mg
- ✓ Cholesterol: 6mg
- ✓ Saturated Fat: 2g

Air Fryer Meatball Subs

Time for Preparation: Ten min.

Time for Cooking: Fifteen min.

Servings: Two-Four

Ingredients:

- 12-16 meatballs (store-bought or homemade)
- Tomato sauce two cups.
- To taste, add salt and pepper.
- Garlic powder half tsp.
- Dried basil Half tsp.
- Dried oregano Half tsp.
- Two-four sub rolls.
- Half cup shredded mozzarella cheese.

Directions:

1. Set the temperature of your air fryer at 400°F (200°C).
2. In a bowl, combine tomato sauce, oregano, basil, pepper, salt, and garlic powder.
3. Insert the basket of air fryer with meatballs, and air fried for 5 minutes.
4. After coating the meatballs with the tomato sauce mixture, air fried them for an additional 5 to 7 mints, or until they are well cooked.

5. Split the bottom roll in half, and then arrange the halves cut-side up in the air fryer basket. The side rolls should be gently browned after 2 to 3 minutes of frying.

6. Remove bottom roll from air fryer and stuff with meatballs and sauce.

7. Sprinkle grated mozzarella cheese over meatballs and sauce.

8. Place the bottom rolls back in the air fryer and cook for a further two to three min or till the cheese is bubbling and melted.

Nutrition:

- ✓ Calories: 477
- ✓ Saturated Fat: 9g
- ✓ Total Fat: 22g
- ✓ Cholesterol: 82mg
- ✓ Protein: 26g
- ✓ Dietary Fiber: 4g
- ✓ Total Carbohydrate: 44g
- ✓ Sodium: 1196mg
- ✓ Sugar: 9g

Air Fryer Fried Rice

Time for Preparation: 10 min.

Time for Cooking: 15 min.

Servings: 2-4

Ingredients:

- cooked rice two cups.
- Half cup diced carrots
- Frozen peas half cup.
- Sesame oil one tsp.
- Vegetable oil one tbsp.
- Diced onion half cup.
- Two tbsp. soy sauce

- Two cloves garlic, minced
- 2 eggs, beaten
- Green onions, chopped as a garnish (optional)
- To taste, add black pepper and salt.

Directions:

1. Set the air fryer to 200 °C.

2. Combine cooked rice, carrots, peas, onions and garlic in a bowl.

3. Stir-fry the rice mixture in the basket of air fryer for five minutes at a time or until the veggies are just beginning to soften.

4. In another bowl, mix soy sauce, salad oil, and sesame oil.

5. 5. Put the beaten eggs in the basket of air fryer and cook for a further 2 to 3 min, till they are fully cooked.

6. Pour the combined soy sauce over the mixed rice in the air fryer basket.

7. Air fried the rice until it is somewhat crispy for 5-7 minutes, tossing every 2-3 minutes.

8. Stir the rice and cooked egg together. Add salt and pepper to taste.

9. 9. If preferred, add minced green onions as a garnish.

Nutrition:

- ✓ Calories: 232
- ✓ Protein: 8g
- ✓ Sugar: 3g
- ✓ Dietary Fiber: 3g
- ✓ Total Carbohydrate: 30g
- ✓ Sodium: 558mg
- ✓ Cholesterol: 93mg
- ✓ Saturated Fat: 2g

✓ Total Fat: 9g

Air Fryer Coconut Chicken

Time for Preparation: Ten min.

Time for Cooking: Fifteen min.

Servings: 2-4

Ingredients:

- 1 lb. of shredded skinless, boneless chicken breast
- Half tsp. paprika
- Garlic powder Half tsp.
- Black pepper 1/4 tsp.
- All-purpose flour Half cup.
- Salt Half tsp.
- One beaten egg
- Half cup shredded coconut

Directions:

1. Set air fryer to 190°C before using.
2. Add flour, garlic powder, black pepper, salt, and paprika to a basin and mix.
3. In another dish, beat the eggs.
4. Make sure that each chicken strip is thoroughly coated before dredging it in the flour mixture, beaten egg, and coconut flakes.
5. Arrange the chicken strips in a single layer in the basket of air fryer. Cook the chicken for ten to twelve min, or until it is well cooked, and the coconut shell is crisp and golden.

Nutrition:

- ✓ Calories: 306
- ✓ Protein: 33g
- ✓ Dietary Fiber: 3g

✓ Total Carbohydrate: 14g

✓ Sodium: 461mg

✓ Cholesterol: 129mg

✓ Saturated Fat: 8g

✓ Total Fat: 13g

✓ Sugar: 2g

Air Fryer Falafel Pitas

Time for Preparation: 20 min.

Time for Cooking: 15 min.

Servings: Two-Four

Ingredients:

- 1 can chickpeas rinsed and drained.
- Half small onion, roughly chopped
- Minced garlic two cloves.
- Ground coriander one tsp.
- Ground cumin one tsp.
- Fresh cilantro leaves 1/4 cup.
- Fresh parsley leaves 1/4 cup.
- Olive oil 1 tbsp.
- 2 tbsp. all-purpose flour
- Half tsp. salt
- 4 pita breads, warmed
- Toppings of your choice (e.g. hummus, tzatziki, chopped tomatoes, sliced cucumbers)

Directions:

1. The chickpeas, onion, garlic, parsley, cilantro, cumin, coriander and salt should be finely crushed in the food processor.
2. To the mixture in a big bowl, add the flour and the olive oil, and whisk to combine.
3. Set your air fryer's temperature to 375°F. (190°C).

4. Make 16 little patties out of the chickpea mixture.

5. 5. Coat the air fryer basket with nonstick cooking spray before placing the meatballs in one layer. Cooking in batches can be necessary based on the capacity of your air fryer.

6. Air fried the patties for 12 to 15 minutes, turning them over halfway through, or until the outsides are crisp and golden brown.

7. Warm the pita breads on a grill pan or in a toaster oven while the falafel cooks.

8. To construct the pitas, stuff each one with four falafel patties and then add the toppings of your choice.

Nutrition

- ✓ Calories: 315
- ✓ Fiber: 10g
- ✓ Carbohydrates: 52g
- ✓ Cholesterol: 0mg
- ✓ Saturated Fat: 1g
- ✓ Fat: 7g
- ✓ Sugar: 3g
- ✓ Protein: 12g
- ✓ Sodium: 653mg

Air Fryer Chicken Nuggets

Time for Preparation: fifteen min.

Time for Cooking: ten-twelve min.

Servings: two-four

Ingredients:

- 1 pound of chopped bite-sized chicken breast that is skinless and boneless.
- Half cup all-purpose flour.

- Black pepper 1/4 tsp.
- Salt Half tsp.
- Paprika Half tsp.
- Garlic powder Half tsp.
- Onion powder Half tsp.
- Panko breadcrumbs one cup.
- One large beaten egg.
- Cooking spray

Directions:

1. Flour, panko breadcrumbs, garlic powder, black pepper, salt, onion powder, and paprika should be combined in a small bowl.

2. In another little bowl, beat the egg.

3. Flour, garlic, paprika, onion, salt, and black pepper should be combined in a small bowl.

4. In a different little bowl, batter the egg.

5. A third shallow bowl should contain the panko breadcrumbs.

6. Shake off any extra seasoned flour before covering each piece of chicken.

7. After coating the chicken in the panko breadcrumbs, dip it in the beaten egg. Press the breadcrumbs onto the chicken to help them stick.

8. Set your air fryer's temperature to 400°F (205°C).

9. After being sprayed with cooking spray, the chicken nuggets should be placed in the basket of air fryer in a single layer.

10. The chicken nuggets should be air-fried for 10 to 12 minutes, turning them over halfway through, until they are well cooked and golden brown.

11. Hot chicken nuggets should be served with your preferred dipping sauce.

Nutrition

- ✓ Calories: 210
- ✓ Protein: 25g
- ✓ Fiber: 1g
- ✓ Carbohydrates: 16g
- ✓ Cholesterol: 101mg
- ✓ Saturated Fat: 1g
- ✓ Fat: 5g
- ✓ Sugar: 1g
- ✓ Sodium: 504mg

Air Fryer Salmon with Roasted Vegetables

Time for Preparation: 10 min.

Time for Cooking: 12-15 min.

Servings: 2-4

Ingredients:

- 4 salmon fillets, skin removed
- 2 cups mixed vegetables (such as bell peppers, zucchini, and cherry tomatoes), chopped
- 1 lemon, sliced
- 1/4 tsp. black pepper
- Olive oil two tbsp.
- Salt half tsp.
- Cooking spray

Directions:

1. Mix the black pepper, salt, and olive oil with the chopped veggies.

2. Set your air fryer's temperature to 400°F (205°C).

3. After being coated with cooking spray, the salmon fillets should be put in the basket of air fryer in a single layer.

4. Place the seasoned vegetables all around the salmon fillets.

5. Top each salmon fillet with a lemon wedge.

6. Air fried the salmon for twelve to fifteen minutes at a time, or until it is cooked through, and roast the veggies to your preference.

7. Serve hot.

Nutrition

- ✓ Calories: 321
- ✓ Protein: 29g
- ✓ Sugar: 4g
- ✓ Fiber: 4g
- ✓ Carbohydrates: 11g
- ✓ Cholesterol: 78mg
- ✓ Saturated Fat: 3g
- ✓ Fat: 18g
- ✓ Sodium: 367mg

Air Fryer Zucchini Fritters

Time for Preparation: 10 min.

Time for Cooking: 10 min.

Servings: two-four

Ingredients:

- 2 medium-sized zucchinis, grated
- Onion powder 1/4 tsp.
- Grated Parmesan cheese 1/4 cup.
- Garlic powder 1/4 tsp.
- All-purpose flour 1/4 cup.

- To taste, add black pepper and salt.
- 1 large egg
- Cooking spray

Directions:

1. Set the temperature of the air fryer to 375°F (190°C).
2. Combine the grated zucchini, all-purpose flour, garlic powder, onion powder, salt, pepper and Parmesan cheese in a large basin. Mix well.
3. Add the egg to the combination of zucchini and whisk to incorporate.
4. Cooking spray should be used on the air fryer basket.
5. Use a spoon to scoop the zucchini mixture and form it into small fritters.
6. Arrange the fritters in a single layer with room between them in the basket of air fryer.
7. Use frying spray to coat the fritters.
8. Air fried the fritters for five to six min, or till the bottoms are golden brown.
9. Toasted and crispy on both sides, flip the fritters over and air fried for a further five to six minutes on each side.
10. Serve the fritters hot with your favorite dipping sauce.

Nutrition:

- ✓ Calories: 87 kcal
- ✓ Total Fat: 4 g
- ✓ Cholesterol: 54 mg
- ✓ Total Carbohydrate: 8 g
- ✓ Sugar: 1 g
- ✓ Protein: 6 g

- ✓ Fiber: 1 g
- ✓ Saturated Fat: 2 g
- ✓ Sodium: 168 mg

Air Fryer Lemon Garlic Shrimp

Time for Preparation: 10 min.

Time for Cooking: 8 min.

Servings: two-four

Ingredients:

- One lb. large shrimp, deveined and peeled
- Two tbsp. olive oil
- One lemon, juiced.
- Minced garlic two cloves
- To taste, add black pepper and salt.
- Chopped fresh parsley one tbsp.

Directions:

1. Set the air fryer's temperature to 400°F (200°C).
2. Combine the black pepper, salt, lemon juice, chopped garlic, and olive oil in a bowl.
3. Place the prawns in a dish and thoroughly coat them.
4. Arrange the prawns in the basket of the air fryer in a single layer.
5. Air fried the prawns for 4 minutes, then flips them over and cooks for an additional 4 minutes, or until done.
6. Serve the prawns right away after adding some parsley to it.

Nutrition:

- ✓ Calories: 168 kcal
- ✓ Protein: 23 g
- ✓ Saturated Fat: 1 g
- ✓ Cholesterol: 239 mg

- ✓ Total Carbohydrate: 3 g
- ✓ Fiber: 1 g
- ✓ Sugar: 1 g
- ✓ Total Fat: 7 g
- ✓ Sodium: 601 mg

FRUIT AND DESERT RECIPES

Chia and Berries Smoothie Bowl

Preparation Time: 5 minutes

Cooking Time: 0 minutes

Servings: 2

Ingredients:

- 1 and ½ cup almond milk
- 1 cup blackberries
- ¼ cup strawberries, chopped
- 1 and ½ tablespoons chia seeds
- 1 teaspoon cinnamon powder

Directions:

1. In a blender, combine the blackberries with the strawberries and the rest of the ingredients, pulse well, divide into small bowls and serve cold.

Nutrition:

- ✓ Calories 182
- ✓ Fat 3.4g
- ✓ Fiber 3.4 g
- ✓ Carbs 8.4g
- ✓ Protein 3g

Almond Butter Smoothies

Preparation Time: 5 minutes

Cooking Time: 0 minutes

Servings: 1

Ingredients:

- 1 scoop of hemp protein
- 1 Tablespoon natural almond butter
- 1 cup of hemp milk
- 1 banana, preferably frozen for a creamier shake
- few ice cubes

Directions:

1. Blend all ingredients together and enjoy!

Nutrition:

- ✓ Calories: 533 kcal
- ✓ Protein: 31.23 g
- ✓ Fat: 26.31 g
- ✓ Carbohydrates: 47.13 g

Blended Coconut Milk and Banana Breakfast Smoothie

Preparation Time: 10 minutes

Cooking Time: 0 minutes

Servings: 4

Ingredients:

- 4 ripe medium-sized bananas
- 4 tbsp. flax seeds
- 2 cups almond milk
- 2 cups coconut milk
- 4 tsp. cinnamon

Directions:

1. Peel the banana and slice it into ½-inch pieces. Put all the ingredients in the blender and blend into a smoothie.
2. Add a dash of cinnamon at the top of the smoothie before serving.

Nutrition:

- ✓ Calories: 332 kcal
- ✓ Protein: 12.49 g
- ✓ Fat: 14.42 g
- ✓ Carbohydrates: 42.46 g

Kale Smoothie

Preparation Time: 10 minutes

Cooking Time: 0 minutes

Servings: 2

Ingredients:

- 10 kale leaves
- 5 bananas, peeled and cut into chunks
- 2 pears, chopped
- 5 tbsp. almond butter
- 5 cups almond milk

Directions:

1. In your blender, mix the kale with the bananas, pears, almond butter, and almond milk.
2. Pulse well, divide into glasses, and serve. Enjoy!

Nutrition:

- ✓ Calories: 267
- ✓ Fat: 11 g
- ✓ Protein: 7 g
- ✓ Carbs: 15 g
- ✓ Fiber: 7 g

Raspberry Smoothie

Preparation Time: 10 minutes

Cooking Time: 0 minutes

Servings: 2

Ingredients:

- 1 avocado, pitted and peeled
- 3/4 cup raspberry juice
- 3/4 cup orange juice
- 1/2 cup raspberries

Directions:

1. In your blender, mix the avocado with the raspberry juice, orange juice, and raspberries.
2. Pulse well, divide into 2 glasses, and serve. Enjoy!

Nutrition:

- ✓ Calories: 125
- ✓ Fat: 11 g
- ✓ Protein: 3 g
- ✓ Carbs: 9 g
- ✓ Fiber: 7 g

Pineapple Smoothie

Preparation Time: 10 minutes

Cooking Time: 0 minutes

Servings: 2

Ingredients:

- 1 cup coconut water
- 1 orange, peeled and cut into quarters

- 1 1/2 cups pineapple chunks
- 1 tbsp. fresh grated ginger
- 1 tsp. chia seeds
- 1 tsp. turmeric powder
- A pinch black pepper

Directions:

1. In your blender, mix the coconut water with the orange, pineapple, ginger, chia seeds, turmeric, and black pepper.
2. Pulse well, pour into a glass.
3. Serve for breakfast. Enjoy!

Nutrition:

- ✓ Calories: 151
- ✓ Fat: 2 g
- ✓ Protein: 4 g
- ✓ Carbs: 12 g
- ✓ Fiber: 6 g

Beet Smoothie

Preparation Time: 10 minutes

Cooking Time: 0 minutes

Servings: 2

Ingredients:

- 10 oz. almond milk, unsweetened
- 2 beets, peeled and quartered
- 1/2 banana, peeled and frozen
- 1/2 cup cherries, pitted
- 1 tbsp. almond butter

Directions:

1. In your blender, mix the milk with the beets, banana, cherries, and butter.
2. Pulse well, pour into glasses, and serve. Enjoy!

Nutrition:

- ✓ Calories: 165
- ✓ Fat: 5 g
- ✓ Protein: 5 g
- ✓ Carbs: 22 g
- ✓ Fiber: 6 g

Blueberry Smoothie

Preparation Time: 10 minutes

Cooking Time: 0 minutes

Servings: 1

Ingredients:

- 1 banana, peeled
- 2 handfuls baby spinach
- 1 tbsp. almond butter
- 1/2 cup blueberries
- 1/4 tsp. ground cinnamon
- 1 tsp. maca powder
- 1/2 cup water
- 1/2 cup almond milk, unsweetened

Directions:

1. In your blender, mix the spinach with the banana, blueberries, almond butter, cinnamon, maca powder, water, and milk.
2. Pulse well, pour into a glass, and serve. Enjoy!

Nutrition:

- ✓ Calories: 341
- ✓ Fat: 12 g
- ✓ Protein: 10 g
- ✓ Carbs: 54 g
- ✓ Fiber: 12 g

Strawberry Oatmeal Smoothie

Preparation Time: 10 minutes

Cooking Time: 0 minutes

Servings: 1

Ingredients:

- 1 cup soy milk
- 1/2 cup rolled oats
- 1 banana, broken into chunks
- 14 frozen strawberries
- 1/2 tsp. vanilla extract
- 1 1/2 tsp. honey

Directions:

1. Add everything to a blender jug.
2. Cover the jug tightly.
3. Blend until smooth. Serve and enjoy!

Nutrition:

- ✓ Calories: 172
- ✓ Fat: 0.4 g
- ✓ Protein: 5.6 g
- ✓ Carbs: 8 g
- ✓ Fiber: 2 g

Almond Blueberry Smoothie

Preparation Time: 10 minutes

Cooking Time: 0 minutes

Servings: 1

Ingredients:

- 1 cup frozen blueberries
- 1 banana
- 1/2 cup almond milk
- 1 tbsp. almond butter
- Water, as needed

Directions:

1. Add everything to a blender jug.
2. Cover the jug tightly.
3. Blend until smooth. Serve and enjoy!

Nutrition:

- ✓ Calories: 211
- ✓ Fat: 0.2 g
- ✓ Protein: 5.6 g
- ✓ Carbs: 3.4 g
- ✓ Fiber: 2.3 g

Raspberry Banana Smoothie

Preparation Time: 10 minutes

Cooking Time: 0 minutes

Servings: 1

Ingredients:

- 1 banana
- 16 whole almonds
- 1/4 cup rolled oats
- 1 tbsp. flaxseed meal
- 1 cup frozen raspberries
- 1 cup raspberry yogurt
- 1/4 cup Concord grape juice
- 1 cup almond milk

Directions:

1. Add everything to a blender jug.
2. Cover the jug tightly.
3. Blend until smooth and then serve. Enjoy!

Nutrition:

- ✓ Calories: 214
- ✓ Fat: 0.4 g
- ✓ Protein: 5.6 g
- ✓ Carbs: 8 g
- ✓ Fiber: 2.3 g

Avocado Chia Parfait

Preparation Time: 5 minutes

Cooking Time: 20 minutes

Servings: 2

Ingredients:

- 1 tablespoon cashew nuts, chopped
- For the Avocado Jam
- 2 avocados, diced
- 2 tablespoons chia seeds
- ⅛ teaspoon nutmeg powder
- ¾ teaspoon cinnamon powder
- Pinch of sea salt
- For the Parfait Base
- 1¼ cups almond milk
- 1 banana, mashed
- ⅛ teaspoon nutmeg powder
- ½ teaspoon cinnamon powder
- 2 tablespoons pumpkin seeds

Directions:

1. In a bowl, combine almond milk, banana, nutmeg powder, cinnamon powder, and pumpkin seeds. Mix until well combined. Chill in the fridge.
2. Meanwhile, place the saucepan on medium heat. Combine avocados, nutmeg powder, cinnamon powder, and salt. Bring to a boil. Allow simmering for 20 minutes.
3. Turn off the heat. Mash half of the jam using a wooden spoon. Let cool. Set aside.
4. Spoon 2 tablespoons of parfait base and apple jam into parfait glasses. Garnish with cashew nuts. Serve.

Nutrition:

- ✓ Calories: 671 kcal
- ✓ Protein: 13.13 g

- ✓ Fat: 54.86 g
- ✓ Carbohydrates: 43.76 g

Pure Avocado Pudding

Preparation Time: 3 hours

Cooking Time: 0 minutes

Servings: 4

Ingredients:

- 1 cup almond milk
- 2 avocados, peeled and pitted
- ¾ cup cocoa powder
- 1 teaspoon vanilla extract
- 2 tablespoons stevia
- ¼ teaspoon cinnamon
- Walnuts, chopped for serving

Directions:

1. Add avocados to a blender and pulse well
2. Add cocoa powder, almond milk, stevia, vanilla bean extract and pulse the mixture well
3. Place into serving bowls then top with walnuts
4. Chill for 2-3 hours and serve!

Nutrition:

- ✓ Calories: 221
- ✓ Fat: 8g
- ✓ Carbohydrates: 7g
- ✓ Protein: 3g

Sweet Almond and Coconut Fat Bombs

Preparation Time: 10 minutes + 20 minutes chill time

Cooking Time: 0 minutes

Servings: 4

Ingredients:

- ¼ cup melted coconut oil
- 9 and ½ tablespoons almond butter
- 90 drops liquid stevia
- 3 tablespoons cocoa
- 9 tablespoons melted almond butter, sunflower seeds

Directions:

1. Take a bowl and add all of the listed ingredients
2. Mix them well
3. Pour scant 2 tablespoons of the mixture into as many muffin molds as you like
4. Chill for 20 minutes and pop them out
5. Serve and enjoy!

Nutrition:

- ✓ Total Carbs: 2g
- ✓ Fiber: 0g
- ✓ Protein: 2.53g
- ✓ Fat: 14g

60 DAYS MEAL PLAN

DAYS	BREAKFAST	LUNCH	DINNER
1	WILD RICE, CELERY, AND CAULIFLOWER PILAF	MINESTRONE CHICKPEAS AND MACARONI CASSEROLE	SMALL PASTA AND BEANS POT
2	ISRAELI EGGPLANT, CHICKPEA, AND MINT SAUTÉ	SLOW COOKED TURKEY AND BROWN RICE	ITALIAN BAKED BEANS
3	BROWN RICE PILAF WITH PISTACHIOS AND RAISINS	PAPAYA, JICAMA, AND PEAS RICE BOWL	CANNELLINI BEAN LETTUCE WRAPS
4	CHERRY, APRICOT, AND PECAN BROWN RICE BOWL	ITALIAN BAKED BEANS	SPICY KINGFISH
5	LEBANESE FLAVOR BROKEN THIN NOODLES	CANNELLINI BEAN LETTUCE WRAPS	CURRY APPLE COUSCOUS WITH LEEKS AND PECANS
6	FARROTTO MIX	LENTILS AND RICE	LEBANESE FLAVOR BROKEN THIN NOODLES
7	FETA-GRAPE-BULGUR SALAD WITH GRAPES AND FETA	CURRY APPLE COUSCOUS WITH LEEKS AND PECANS	LEMONY FARRO AND AVOCADO BOWL
8	GREEK STYLE MEATY BULGUR	LEMONY FARRO AND AVOCADO BOWL	RICE AND BLUEBERRY STUFFED SWEET POTATOES
9	HEARTY BARLEY MIX	RICE AND BLUEBERRY STUFFED SWEET POTATOES	DILL HADDOCK
10	HEARTY BARLEY RISOTTO	CURRY CHICKEN LETTUCE WRAPS	GINGERED TILAPIA
11	HEARTY FREEKEH PILAF	NACHO CHICKEN CASSEROLE	HADDOCK WITH SWISS CHARD
12	HERBY-LEMONY FARRO	PESTO & MOZZARELLA CHICKEN CASSEROLE	CODFISH STICKS
13	MUSHROOM-BULGUR PILAF	CHICKEN QUICHE	BASMATI RICE PILAF MIX
14	BAKED BROWN RICE	CHICKEN PARMIGIANA	TASTY SPRING SALAD
15	BARLEY PILAF	BAKED CHICKEN MEATBALLS - HABANERO & GREEN CHILI	TOASTED CUMIN CRUNCH
16	BASMATI RICE PILAF MIX	WINTER CHICKEN WITH VEGETABLES	HALIBUT STIR FRY
17	BROWN RICE SALAD WITH ASPARAGUS, GOAT CHEESE, AND LEMON	PAPRIKA CHICKEN & PANCETTA IN A SKILLET	WINTER CHICKEN WITH VEGETABLES
18	CARROT-ALMOND-BULGUR SALAD	PULLED BUFFALO CHICKEN SALAD WITH BLUE CHEESE	CHICKEN CAPRESE
19	CHICKPEA-SPINACH-BULGUR	RED PEPPER AND MOZZARELLA-STUFFED CHICKEN CAPRESE	TOMATO-BASIL SAUCE
20	GREEK FARRO SALAD	CHILI & LEMON MARINATED CHICKEN WINGS	WHOLE-WHEAT PASTA WITH
21	PURE DELISH SPINACH SALAD	GREEK STYLE MEATY BULGUR	LENTILS WITH TOMATOES AND TURMERIC
22	TENDER CREAMY SCALLOPS.	RICE AND BLUEBERRY STUFFED SWEET POTATOES	PULLED BUFFALO CHICKEN SALAD WITH BLUE CHEESE
23	SALMON BALLS	FETA-GRAPE-BULGUR SALAD WITH GRAPES AND FETA	RED PEPPER AND MOZZARELLA-STUFFED

24	FRIED CODFISH WITH ALMONDS	CARROT-ALMOND-BULGUR SALAD	PAPRIKA CHICKEN & PANCETTA IN A SKILLET
25	OVEN-BAKED SOLE FILLETS	CHICKPEA-SPINACH-BULGUR	CHILI & LEMON MARINATED CHICKEN WINGS
26	GRILLED SALMON WITH CAPONATA	TARRAGON CHICKEN WITH ROASTED BALSAMIC TURNIPS	CIPOLLINI & BELL PEPPER CHICKEN SOUVLAKI
27	QUICK SHRIMP MOQUECA	TURMERIC CHICKEN WINGS WITH GINGER SAUCE	TOASTED CUMIN CRUNCH
28	THAI CHOWDER	CURRY CHICKEN LETTUCE WRAPS	LIGHT MUSHROOM RISOTTO
29	HERBED ROCKFISH	NACHO CHICKEN CASSEROLE	VEGETABLE PIE
30	COCONUT RICE WITH SHRIMPS IN COCONUT CURRY	BAKED CHICKEN MEATBALLS - HABANERO & GREEN CHILI	TURMERIC NACHOS
31	WASABI SALMON BURGERS	WINTER CHICKEN WITH VEGETABLES	RUCOLA SALAD
32	NUT-CRUST TILAPIA WITH KALE	PAPRIKA CHICKEN & PANCETTA IN A SKILLET	TASTY SPRING SALAD
33	EASY CRUNCHY FISH TRAY BAKE	PULLED BUFFALO CHICKEN SALAD WITH BLUE CHEESE	GREEK STYLE MEATY BULGUR
34	COD CURRY	CHILI & LEMON MARINATED CHICKEN WINGS	HEARTY BARLEY MIX
35	GINGER SALMON AND BLACK BEANS	CIPOLLINI & BELL PEPPER CHICKEN SOUVLAKI	HEARTY BARLEY RISOTTO
36	HONEY CRUSTED SALMON WITH PECANS	TURNIP GREENS & ARTICHOKE CHICKEN	BAKED BROWN RICE
37	SALMON CAKES	LENTILS WITH TOMATOES AND TURMERIC	MUSHROOM-BULGUR PILAF
38	ORANGE AND MAPLE-GLAZED SALMON	WHOLE-WHEAT PASTA WITH TOMATO-BASIL SAUCE	TURNIP GREENS & ARTICHOKE CHICKEN
39	QUICK COLLARD GREENS	NUTTY AND FRUITY GARDEN SALAD	HEARTY FREEKEH PILAF
40	MANHATTAN-STYLE SALMON CHOWDER	ROASTED ROOT VEGETABLES	LEBANESE FLAVOR
41	ROASTED SALMON AND ASPARAGUS	BRAISED KALE	HERBY-LEMONY FARRO
42	CITRUS SALMON ON A BED OF GREENS	BRAISED LEEKS, CAULIFLOWER AND ARTICHOKE HEARTS	STUFFED SWEET POTATOES
43	WILD RICE WITH SPICY CHICKPEAS	CELERY ROOT HASH BROWNS	CHERRY, APRICOT, AND PECAN BROWN RICE BOWL
44	CASHEW PESTO & PARSLEY WITH VEGGIES	BRAISED CARROTS 'N KALE	CURRY APPLE COUSCOUS WITH LEEKS AND PECANS
45	SPICY CHICKPEAS WITH ROASTED VEGETABLES	CAULIFLOWER FRITTERS	ASPARAGUS WITH GARLIC
46	VEGETABLE AND EGG CASSEROLE	SWEET POTATO PUREE	AVOCADO TOMATO SALAD
47	TOFU SPINACH SAUTÉ	VEGETABLE POTPIE	ZUCCHINI RAVIOLI

48	MEXICAN CAULIFLOWER RICE	TASTY SPRING SALAD	CAULIFLOWER SALAD
49	VEGETABLE PIE	SPECIAL VEGETABLE KITCHREE	TOFU SPINACH SAUTÉ
50	RUCOLA SALAD	MASHED SWEET POTATO BURRITOS	VEGETABLE AND EGG CASSEROLE
51	BLACK EYED-PEAS CURRY	TOASTED CUMIN CRUNCH	GREEN BUDDHA BOWL
52	VEGAN MEATBALLS	LIGHT MUSHROOM RISOTTO	SPAGHETTI SQUASH
53	CAULIFLOWER FRITTERS	VEGETABLE PIE	ROASTED GREEN BEANS AND MUSHROOMS
54	PURE AVOCADO PUDDING	TURMERIC NACHOS	ROSEMARY-LEMON COD
55	VEGETABLE PIE	LEMONY FARRO AND AVOCADO BOWL	SALMON WITH MUSTARD CREAM
56	GREEN BUDDHA BOWL	BROWN RICE PILAF WITH PISTACHIOS AND RAISINS	BLACKENED FISH TACOS WITH SLAW
57	AVOCADO CHAI PARFAIT	CURRY APPLE COUSCOUS WITH LEEKS AND PECANS	TILAPIA WITH PARMESAN BARK
58	AVOCADO TOMATO SALAD	MUSHROOM-BULGUR PILAF	STEAMED GARLIC-DILL HALIBUT
59	PAPAYA, JICAMA, AND PEAS RICE BOWL	CASHEW PESTO & PARSLEY WITH VEGGIES	GINGER & CHILI SEA BASS FILLETS
60	NUTTY AND FRUITY GARDEN SALAD	SPICY CHICKPEAS WITH ROASTED VEGETABLES	CITRUS & HERB SARDINES

GET YOUR BONUSES NOW
↓ Exercise for a stronger heart and Anti-Inflammatory Diet↓

OR

CLICK HERE

CONCLUSION

I sincerely appreciate each of you reading my cookbook about heart health. Sharing my love of cooking with you makes me feel honoured. I sincerely hope you enjoyed this cookbook and learned something from the information and dishes included.

The heart-healthy cookbook has immense value for individuals searching to improve their health and fitness. It provides a wealth of information about the benefits of a heart-healthy diet and practical and delicious recipes that can be easily incorporated into your daily routine. Whether trying to prevent heart disease, manage an existing condition, or maintain a healthy lifestyle, this cookbook is a valuable resource to help you achieve your goals.

Please study this cookbook carefully, learn the dishes, and start incorporating heart-healthy practices into your daily life to get the most out of it. Whether you cook one recipe per week or try a new recipe every day, I encourage you to be creative, have fun, and experiment with fresh ingredients and flavour combinations. By following a heart-healthy diet and making healthy cooking a regular part of your life, you can enjoy all the benefits of a healthier heart.

If you want to improve your heart health and lower your risk of heart disease, go through the heart-healthy diet in this cookbook. Readers are exposed to various foods and meals high in fibre, minerals, and healthy fats yet low in sodium, cholesterol, and saturated and trans fats.

Key Points and Takeaways:

The significance of a heart-healthy diet: If you want to lower your risk of heart disease and improve your cardiovascular health overall, eating a heart-healthy diet is crucial. Blood pressure, cholesterol, and weight maintenance can all be enhanced with a heart-healthy diet.

Foods to avoid: Certain foods should be avoided or limited to maintaining a healthy heart, including processed and packaged foods, red meat, fried foods, sugary drinks, processed snacks, butter and margarine, high-fat dairy products, and baked goods.

Foods to eat: A heart-healthy diet should include a wide variety of whole foods, including fruits and vegetables; lean proteins like fish, poultry, and legumes, including pulses; beneficial fats like oil from olives as well as nuts, including low-fat or fat-free dairy goods.

Healthy cooking methods: Healthy cooking methods like baking, broiling, grilling, and steaming can help reduce the intake of unhealthy fats and calories.

Incorporating healthy habits: Besides adopting a heart-healthy diet, healthy habits like regular exercise, stress management, and getting enough sleep can also improve heart health.

Maintaining a healthy heart and reducing the risk of heart disease can be accomplished by adopting a heart-friendly diet. Fresh, whole foods are emphasized in the heart-healthy diet because they are abundant in fibre, minerals, and good fats while being low in salt, cholesterol, saturated fats, and trans fats. A heart-healthy diet can help lower the risk of heart problems by lowering blood pressure and cholesterol, particularly the body mass index. (BMI).

Making healthy changes can be difficult, but it is essential to remember that small changes can add up over time. The heart-healthy cookbook provides readers with a wide range of recipes and meal ideas that are both nutritious and delicious, making it easier to adopt a heart-healthy diet. Additionally, the cookbook offers practical tips and advice for incorporating healthy habits into everyday life, such as setting goals, meal planning, and staying motivated.

We want to inform you that these recipes are more superficial than most other diet plans because of the simple dishes. If you don't have time to cook everything right immediately, there are several various recipes you can utilize. Several recipes don't require unusual ingredients because you can usually make them with cupboard staples.

In conclusion, adopting a heart-healthy diet can provide numerous benefits for overall health and well-being, including a reduced risk of heart disease, improved weight management, better blood sugar control, increased nutrient intake, improved mood and mental health, and a lower risk of other chronic diseases. Reading this heart-healthy cookbook can provide valuable guidance and support for making healthier food choices and preparing delicious, heart-healthy meals. One's cardiovascular health can be improved, and their risk of heart disease can be decreased by making minor, lasting modifications to their diet. Individuals can take the first step toward a healthier and happier life with the support and guidance provided in this heart-healthy cookbook.

I also want to remind you that the information in this cookbook is not a substitute for medical advice. Always visit your doctor if you have any concerns regarding your health. However, this heart-healthy cookbook has taught you how to alter your lifestyle and what foods to eat to prevent many of the most prevalent heart issues of the present. Anyone trying to enhance their lifestyle and health should consider it.

MEASUREMENT CONVERSION CHART

Temperature Conversions:

Celsius	Fahrenheit
0°C	32°F
100°C	212°F
150°C	302°F
180°C	356°F
200°C	392°F
220°C	428°F
250°C	482°F

Weight Conversions:

Metric	Imperial	US Customary
1 gram	0.035 oz.	0.04 oz.
100 grams	3.5 oz.	3.5 oz.
250 grams	8.8 oz.	8.8 oz.
500 grams	1.1 lb.	1.1 lb.
1 kg	2.2 lb.	2.2 lb.

Volume Conversions:

Metric	Imperial	US Customary
1 ml	0.03 FL oz.	0.03 FL oz.
100 ml	3.4 FL oz.	3.4 FL oz.
250 ml	8.5 FL oz.	8.5 FL oz.
500 ml	17 FL oz.	2.1 cups
1 liter	1.8 pints	4.2 cups

Made in the USA
Las Vegas, NV
03 November 2023

80148190R00050